PERFECT *FIT*

WEEKLY **WISDOM** & **WORKOUTS** FOR WOMEN OF **FAITH** & **FITNESS**

DIANA ANDERSON-TYLER

Red Slippers Press

DISCLAIMER

CONTENTS

INTRODUCTION

Hello, ladies! I hope this book finds you well and ready to refresh your spirit and revitalize your body and soul! It's been two years since my second book, *Fit for Faith: A Christian Woman's Guide to Total Fitness,* was published. Please allow me to update you on my life a bit so you can understand exactly *why* I've written a book with workouts so undeniably different than those I programmed in my first two books. (Believe me, I never thought I'd stray from my old-school routines!)

The spring before *Fit for Faith*'s release, I met my husband Ben at a local community workout my gym was hosting. We were married less than seven months later and opened our very own box seven months after that![1]

---

1   "Box" is CrossFit speak for "gym" because these facilities typically look just like, well, a box—sparsely decorated warehouse-type buildings without the bells and whistles typically seen in workout centers and health clubs.

During the same time I was falling in love with Ben, I was simultaneously becoming more and more infatuated with a method of working out that had previously been foreign to me, something I had never seen before in my years of weight lifting and personal training. It was heart-pumping, sweat-inducing, pride-breaking, boredom-busting, and altogether eye-opening. It was *CrossFit*.

CrossFit is a bit hard to define as it encompasses a wide variety of exercises and modalities that don't exactly fit neatly into a verbal nutshell. To quote Wikipedia, CrossFit "combines weightlifting, sprinting, gymnastics, powerlifting, kettlebell training, plyometrics, rowing, and medicine ball training."

I was quite familiar with the first item, weightlifting, when I began, but had no experience with, nor interest in, for that matter, the remaining seven components. The expressions "Secure in my comfort zone" and "Fear of the unknown" perfectly encapsulated my reservations.

To speedily get you up to speed, CrossFit training has truly molded me into my most fit, most athletic state to date. I remember the first class I took. There were burpees. Lots and lots of burpees. And running, an activity I'd loathed since suicide drills in high school basketball practices. I was immediately smitten with a merciless bolt of humility as I realized: *I'm not as fit as I thought I was!* And the day I saw the words "snatch" and "clean" written on the dry-erase board as part of the workout, I thought they were referencing petty theft and hygiene, *not* Olympic lifts.

In just over a year, I can run a 7:05 mile, burpees don't give me stress-induced acne, and I'm proud to be doing lifts, such as a 265-pound deadlift and bodyweight clean and jerk, that make me hear the "Rocky" theme song.

Those are just a few of the improvements I'm noticing in my physical fitness, and what makes it all the more awesome and enjoyable is the fact that it pleases the Lord and enhances my spiritual fitness as well.

Romans 12:1 proclaims that our bodies are to be a "living and holy sacrifice, the kind He will find acceptable." It makes perfect sense to me that the stronger, fitter, healthier we are, the more "acceptable" our "sacrifice," that is, our bodies. I'm so thankful for the body and health He's given me, and it's my joy to take care of it the best I can and help you do the same.

It's an honor and pleasure to introduce you to a fun, challenging style of training, as well as to some of the incredible women I've had the privilege to meet, pray with, and sweat beside. May you be richly blessed as you read and ponder the following devotionals and testimonies written by women striving for God's best in their lives.

"As iron sharpens iron, so one man sharpens another." ~Proverbs 27:17

In the following pages, you'll find one devotional and two workouts per week. I recommend that you give yourself a day or two between workouts, at least initially. As you become fitter and more accustomed to the intensity of the routines, you may be able to work out on consecutive days. These workouts can supplement your current training routine, or can be easily added onto should you decide to add other workout days to your schedule; other books and online sources can help you program a custom-made at-home workout plan.

Stay fit, stay faithful,

PROLOGUE
WHAT YOU'LL
NEED TO GET YOUR
WORKOUT ON!

Are you ready to get into the best shape of your life and, as we say at CrossFit 925, "discover your inner athlete"?! I hope so! But before we get started, allow me to brief you on the equipment I recommend that you purchase—or pull out of the closet or garage!—to help optimize your workouts.[2] You can locate and/or order any and all of the following equipment online.

Also, before you dive into the workouts, I encourage you to go to my website [http://www.dianafit.com/downloads/] and print out the monthly Workout Logs that are available for you to record the results of every workout, including the weight you used and your time or score.

---

2   The only mandatory equipment is a pair of dumbbells and a kettlebell. Modifications are included in each workout for those of you who don't have and/or don't wish to acquire a pull-up bar or plyo box.

DUMBBELLS

Of course, we all know what dumbbells are, but why have them in our homes? Well, dumbbells are, quite simply, a workout staple. They are the meat to a treadmill's potatoes. They're the Sonny to the bicycle's Cher. And they've withstood the test of time. The word "dumbbell" originated in the sixteenth century when novice church bell ringers found they'd better gain some brawn to do their job adequately. To develop their arm strength, the ringers connected a rope to a metal weight and swung it against imaginary bells which produced no sound, hence, it was a *dumb* bell. In the eighteenth century, "dumb-bells" became the first pieces of home gym equipment, and a hundred years later, the short bar we know today replaced the rope, and rounded weights were attached at either end.

Dumbbells ensure a balanced workout because they effectively train every muscle group. They offer an increased range of motion, guarantee a challenge so you don't plateau, are completely portable, and most importantly, they're affordable.[3]

If you're brand new to weight training, I suggest purchasing a pair of five, eight, and ten pound dumbbells. When the ten pounders become too light, move up to twelve, fifteen, and even twenty pounds.

If you've been lifting weights for a while, I recommend buying weights in five-pound increments, from five pounds up to thirty.

KETTLEBELL

The kettlebell was developed in Russia in the 1700s and used by the Soviet army as part of their physical training (Can you get any more hardcore?). This cannonball-like cast iron device is an incredible tool for developing strength and endurance as each exercise we

3   Info from Diana's book, *Fit for Faith: A Christian Woman's Guide to Total Fitness*

do with it requires the entire body. Here are a few more facts about your new favorite workout partner:

- Full-body conditioning
- Because kettlebell training involves multiple muscle groups and energy systems at once, you'll spend less time working out and still get greater results!
- Increased resistance to injury
- The ability to work aerobically and anaerobically simultaneously[4]
- Improved mobility and range of motion
- Enhanced performance in sports and everyday functioning
- Major calorie burning (In a recent study conducted by the highly respected American Council on Exercise, participants burned approximately 20 calories per minute—that's 1,200 calories per hour.)[5]

I suggest starting out with an 18-pound kettlebell and working up to 35 pounds as you increase your strength in the coming weeks.

PLYO BOX

Plyometrics refers to exercise that enables a muscle to reach maximum force in the shortest possible time. The muscle is loaded with an eccentric (lengthening) action, followed immediately by a concentric action. A few fast facts:

- Power exercises such as plyometrics train both speed and strength, killing two birds with one stone and again, cutting the average workout time in half.

---

4   While "aerobic" means "with oxygen," anaerobic means "without air" or "without oxygen." Anaerobic exercise is short-lasting, high-intensity activity, where your body's demand for oxygen exceeds the oxygen supply available. The American College of Sports Medicine (ACSM) defines aerobic exercise as "any activity that uses large muscle groups, can be maintained continuously, and is rhythmic in nature."

5   http://www.acefitness.org/getfit/studies/Kettlebells012010.pdf

- They involve compound movements, boosting anabolic hormones that literally force your body to store energy as muscle rather than fat.

Plyometrics boxes are nice, but "nice" comes with a hefty price! (For those of you with the tools and know-how—or maybe a husband or boyfriend with the tools and know-how—there are great online guides for helping you build your own!)

If buying or building your own isn't an option, then what you want to look for is something sturdy enough to withstand you jumping on it like a monkey on a trampoline. A low, sturdy table or park bench are two great ideas. A stack of *Glamour* or *Us Weekly* magazines is NOT a good idea!

As for height, the typical plyometrics box is about 20 inches tall, but feel free to tweak this according to your skill and whatever you have on hand. Beginners should start with something lower and then work their way up.

PULL-UP BAR

I highly recommend you invest in a pull-up bar and have one installed in your house or garage. It will let you perform multiple compound movements without occupying a lot of space.[6] The primary exercise you'll be doing on the bar is the simple yet beautiful pull-up, which is one of the best strength-builders and muscle developers around, bar none (pun intended). While several other exercises can be performed on the bar, such as hanging knee raises, toes-to-bar, and knees-to-elbows, I've limited its use to pull-ups for simplicity's sake to accommodate readers who won't have a bar.

Another reason I love the idea of having a pull-up bar in your household is that it's an ever-present motivator! When you don't

---

6   Compound exercises require you to use more than one muscle group and more than one joint when you perform them. These types of exercises recruit a maximal amount of muscle fibers, helping you burn fat and build muscle efficiently.

feel like leaving the house to go to the gym, you can get a great workout in because your buddy the bar is there waiting for you to monkey around on! Even just passing by it in your house or glancing at it as you start your car in the garage in the morning will serve as constant, encouraging reminders of your growing strength as well as your dedication to a fit, healthy lifestyle.

What if I can't do pull-ups? I'm glad you asked! Read on!

RESISTANCE BANDS

Resistance bands are invaluable when it comes to pull-ups, because, let's face it, pull-ups don't come naturally to most people, women especially! The bands provide assistance by helping you rebound more easily from the bottom position so you can pull yourself up to achieve the full range of motion necessary for an effective pull-up.

Choose your band according to its level of resistance and your level of fitness. Bands are color-coded. Yellow offers the least resistance, red offers medium resistance, green greater resistance, and gray the most resistance. As you become stronger, you'll be able to move from greater to least resistance until eventually, if you stick with it, you'll be doing pull-ups like a Navy SEAL! (a very pretty, feminine Navy SEAL.)

Now, how to use them and perform a pull-up![7]

STEP 1: Tie one end of the resistance band to the center of your pull-up bar. Wrap the end around the bar then loop the other end of the resistance band through the top loop and pull down. This firmly connects the band to the bar.

STEP 2: Place one foot halfway inside the bottom of the resistance band as if you were gently standing on the band. Put your other foot, slightly bent, in front of the first foot so your ankles are crossed.

---

7   If you don't have access to a pull-up bar, you'll be using dumbbells to perform either overhanded or underhanded rows.

STEP 3: Grip the pull-up bar on either side of the band with your palms facing outwards, wider than shoulder-width apart.

STEP 4: Pull yourself up while keeping your lower body rigid. Continue pulling until your chin is over the bar.

STEP 5: Slowly lower yourself back down while continuing to grip the bar with your hands. Lower as far to the ground as you can get. Step one foot out carefully, and then the other.

ABMAT

The standard sit-up for which you lie flat on your back limits your range of motion, compresses the spine onto the ground, and places you at a relaxed state between repetitions. The AbMat is a nifty little pad that goes beneath your lower back, right above your waistband, to allow you to complete a sit-up's full range of motion and feel a full stretch.

I personally am a fan of the AbMat because it's comfortable and snug under my back and, unlike a towel or other object, it doesn't slide, wobble, or lose its form. If you don't want to purchase one, I recommend using a tightly rolled-up towel or small, firm pillow instead. Anything to brace your lower back is better than nothing!

WEEK 1

"Praise be to the God and Father of our Lord Jesus Christ! In his great mercy he has given us new birth into a living hope through the resurrection of Jesus Christ from the dead, and into an inheritance that can never perish, spoil or fade..." ~1 Peter 1:3-4, NIV

Well, another year is here! While I could write about resolutions and try my hand at motivating you to start a fresh fitness routine or inspiring you to improve your diet, I'll spare you another New Year's spiel. Instead, I'd like to focus for a moment not on the next twelve months, but on eternity. The Scriptures promise us a great inheritance that includes the "crown of life," "mansions," and great "rewards" for our faithfulness (James 1:12, John 14:2, Matthew 5:12).

One of my favorite C.S. Lewis quotes reminds us that our bodies are merely houses for our souls and spirits: "You don't have a soul. You are a soul. You have a body."

One day, those of us who have accepted Jesus Christ as our Lord will leave these corruptible, immortal tents and meet our Savior face to face where we will dwell with Him and the other saints *forever* (2 Corinthians 5:1)! Until our glorious graduation from life to life everlasting, let it be our pleasure to honor God with our bodies , to eat, to sleep, to train, to serve...all for Him!

This week, as tabloids tout surefire ways to shed unwanted holiday weight and get on the fast track to "Your best butt ever!" or "A sizzling six-pack in sixty days!," just remember that the buns of steel we build and rock-hard abs we sculpt will one day meet the same fate as the glossy magazine pages we so often flip through for advice; to dust we shall return (Genesis 3:19).

In a world increasingly fixated on physical appearances, I encourage you to let the words of Paul below echo in your heart. While this world and everything in it—including our bodies—is fading away, the work we do with them for the glory of God does not.

"Physical training is good, but training for godliness is much better, promising benefits in this life and in the life to come." ~1 Timothy 4:8, NIV

Lord, thank You for creating me "fearfully" and "wonderfully." In light of eternity, I know that this life is just a mist. Until I go to my eternal home, I ask You to supply the strength, discipline, and self-control I need to be a faithful steward of my body. In Jesus' Name, Amen.

WORKOUT 1 — WEEK 1

WARMUP

2 rounds:

- ☐ 20 stationary lunges (10 each leg)
- ☐ 20 stationary butt-kicks (10 each leg)
- ☐ 20 stationary high-knees (10 each leg)
- ☐ 20 high-kicks (10 each leg)
- ☐ 15 air squats
- ☐ 10 push-ups
- ☐ 5 burpees

WORKOUT BENCHMARK WORKOUT

"Perfect Fit Benchmark 1" (Record results in your "Workout Log".)

16 minute AMRAP (as many rounds as possible):

- ☐ 5 pull-ups (Substitute bent-over dumbbell rows if you don't have a pull-up bar with bands to assist you, or you don't have access to a gym with an assisted pull-up machine.)
- ☐ 7 push-ups
- ☐ 9 air squats

WORKOUT 2 — WEEK 1

WARMUP

- ☐ 30 lunges with twist over lunging leg (15 each leg)
- ☐ 30 air squats
- ☐ 10 walk-out/walk-ins
- ☐ 30 jumping jacks
- ☐ 15 jump squats
- ☐ 400-meter run (0.25 miles)[8]

WORKOUT

Complete the following as fast as you can with proper form, in the order given: And don't forget your timer![9]

- ☐ 150 jump rope
- ☐ 100 walking lunges[10]
- ☐ 75 jump rope
- ☐ 50 walking lunges
- ☐ 30 jump rope
- ☐ 25 walking lunges
- ☐ 15 jump rope
- ☐ 12 walking lunges

---

8   If doing the workouts at home, I recommend going outside (as long as it's safe!) and approximating this distance. If you're at the gym, hop on the treadmill!

9   Never forgo proper form and technique for a faster time. Speed and intensity are important, but safety is even more crucial, so slow it down if you feel your form begin to deteriorate.

10   Lunge for a total of 100 reps, not 100 each leg (because that would be crazy!!)

WEEK 2

"He has made everything beautiful in its time. He has also set eternity in the human heart" ~Ecclesiastes 3:11, NIV

Did you catch that? The wisest man ever, Solomon, said God made *everything* beautiful. That means **you**! Whether you're currently overweight, underweight, have crooked teeth, a crooked nose, or struggle with acne-prone skin (raising my hand!), you are still a creation of the Most High God, the One who spoke spiral galaxies into existence, the One who weaves babies together in their mothers' wombs (John 1:1, Psalm 139:13).

Glamour magazines and entertainment news shows may hail one hairstyle or makeup trend as this season's "hottest look," but these fashion fads are just that: fads. While the world's ideas of beauty change with the seasons, God's concept of it is *eternal*. I think—make that *"know"*—it would serve us well to view our outward appearance the way our Maker does: gorgeous, exquisite, wonderfully made, eternally loved (Psalm 119:14, Romans 8:39).

The latter part of today's verse speaks of eternity, where our eternal inheritance is, as last week's verse made clear. As you go about your day today, don't let tabloids, commercials, billboards, or even people surrounding you negatively affect how you view yourself. Remain (or seek to become!) dedicated to a healthy lifestyle that doesn't pursue fitness in order to look a certain way or fit into this winter's preferred skinny jean. Pursue fitness to serve God and bring Him glory with the gifts and responsibilities He's entrusted to you.

Dear Lord, thank You for Your beautiful creation. I know that, as a part of this creation, I too, am beautiful. Help me never to forget this fact. No matter what the world says, no matter how designers and celebrities define "beauty," I pray I always remember that the only One whose opinion matters is Yours. I love You, Father. Amen.

WORKOUT 1 — WEEK 2

WARMUP

2 rounds:

- [ ] 20 butt-kicks (10 each leg)
- [ ] 20 high-knees (10 each leg)
- [ ] 20 mountain-climbers (right/left = 1 rep)
- [ ] 15 air squats
- [ ] 15 push-ups
- [ ] 5 burpees

WORKOUT

Time yourself as you complete the following as fast as you can with proper form:

5 rounds:

- [ ] 15 burpees
- [ ] 10 dumbbell push-press
- [ ] 5 broad jumps

WORKOUT 2 — WEEK 2

WARMUP

3 rounds:

- ☐ 10 reverse lunges (5 each leg)
- ☐ 10 high skips (5 each leg)
- ☐ 10 wall squats
- ☐ 15 mock kettlebell swings

WORKOUT BENCHMARK WORKOUT

"Perfect Fit Benchmark 2" (Record results in your "Workout Log".)

Complete the following in the order given with proper form:

- ☐ Timed 1 mile run
- ☐ *Rest* 1 minute
- ☐ 2 minutes: as many sit-ups as possible
- ☐ *Rest* 1 minute
- ☐ 2 minutes: as many air squats as possible
- ☐ *Rest* 1 minute
- ☐ 2 minutes: as many push-ups as possible[11]

---

11 Push-ups may be performed on your knees if you're unable to do the full range of motion (chest to floor) in standard push-up position.

WEEK 3

"No temptation has seized you except what is common to man. And God is faithful; he will not let you be tempted beyond what you can bear. But when you are tempted, he will also provide a way out so that you can stand up under it." ~1 Corinthians 10:13, NIV

I most commonly associate the word "temptation" with sexual sins, such as lust and marital unfaithfulness. But this verse doesn't limit temptation to just one specific weakness we may face as innate sinners. It's meant to give us strength to face *every* situation in which we find ourselves struggling to stay on the narrow road of righteousness.

In the Greek, the word "temptation" is *peirasmoj* and can be defined as "the condition of things, or a mental state, by which we are enticed to sin."[12] What's intriguing to me about this defini-

12 http://www.biblestudytools.com/lexicons/greek/nas/peirasmos.html (accessed November 12, 2013)

tion is the phrase *mental state.* Having struggled with anorexia and binge-eating disorder during my teen years, I know exactly how it feels to be tempted to under or overeat as a result of what's going on between my ears when emotions run rampant.

Many women, like myself in the past, turn to food for control and comfort during life's storms and trials. (Everyone's heard the saying, "'Desserts' is 'Stressed' spelled backwards!) Whether it's by depriving your body of nutrients, or indulging in unneeded quantities, the temptation to literally feed our pains and anxieties is indeed a sin.

How can the way we eat be sinful, you may ask? Because God's Word makes it clear that everything we do, whether eating or drinking, should all be done for His glory (1 Corinthians 10:31). When we use food as a form of medication, we are *not* glorifying God; quite the opposite, we are *grieving* Him by refusing to ask for and receive His peace, wisdom, and consolation in favor of a short-lived sensory experience.

"Give your burdens to the LORD, and he will take care of you. He will not permit the godly to slip and fall." ~Psalm 55:22 (NLT)

When you have a bad day (not "if," but *when)* and your body and soul are searching for a pick-me-up, don't open the freezer, peek inside the fridge, or raid the pantry for a sweet or salty fix. In reality, munching mindlessly is no "fix" at all, but rather a superficial substitution for the genuine satisfaction supplied by the Holy Spirit.

Remember these words: "…he *will* provide a way out," and go to the Lord with all that is troubling you (1 Corinthians 10:13, emphasis added). I know you will find that the goodness of our Lord is far sweeter than any Sundae, far richer than Dutch chocolate, more addicting than your favorite brand of chips!

"Taste and see that the Lord is good; blessed is the man who takes refuge in Him." ~Psalm 34:8, NIV

Loving Father, we praise You for not leaving us alone in this world to battle temptations in our own strength. We thank You for promising a sure way out if we would simply turn to You and trust You to provide an escape and victory over our every struggle. We ask that, when tribulations come and stress escalates, that You would bring to our remembrance the precious promises of Your inerrant, unfading Word. In Jesus' Name, Amen.

WORKOUT 1 — WEEK 3

WARMUP

- ☐ 400-meter jog
- ☐ 10 walk-out/walk-ins
- ☐ 20 scorpions (10 each side)
- ☐ 20 wall squats
- ☐ 20 sit-ups to toe-reaches
- ☐ 20 jumping jacks

WORKOUT

Complete 21-15-9 reps of the following as fast as you can, maintaining proper form:

- ☐ Suitcase deadlifts with dumbbells[13]
- ☐ Box jumps (20 inches)[14]

AFTERBURN

What's an "Afterburn?" **Glad you asked!** I often like to add a little something special, the "Afterburn," to the end of the day's workout in which athletes give it their all for the last remaining minutes of class, typically either working on a skill or building stamina. Try it out by performing the following:

- ☐ 5 100-meter sprints (0.06 miles), resting ninety seconds between sprints

---

13 Choose a weight that's right for you—not too heavy, not too light! You should start "feeling the burn" at least halfway through the reps.

14 If you don't have a plyometric box available, substitute broad jumps instead.

WORKOUT 2 — WEEK 3

WARMUP

3 rounds:

- [ ] 20 reverse lunges (10 each leg)
- [ ] 20 high-kicks (10 each leg)
- [ ] 5 walk-outs
- [ ] 10 air squats
- [ ] 10 push-ups

WORKOUT

12 min. AMRAP (as many rounds as possible):

- [ ] 200-meter run
- [ ] 10 dumbbell hang-cleans cleans (5 each arm)
- [ ] 10 dumbbell sit-ups

AFTERBURN

- [ ] 100 jump ropes for time

WEEK 4

By	Jill Lang
Age	41
Occupation	Homeschool Mom and CrossFit Coach

"Oh yes, you shaped me first inside, then out; you formed me in my mother's womb. I thank you, High God- you're breathtaking! Body and soul, I am marvelously made! I worship in adoration-what a creation! You know me inside and out, you know every bone in my body; You know exactly how I was made, bit by bit, how I was sculpted from nothing into something. Like an open book, you watched me grow from conception to birth; all the stages of my life were spread out before you, The days of my life all prepared before I'd even lived one day" ~Psalm 139:13-16, MSG

Did you know God is crazy about you?! It's true. He is absolutely desperately in-love with you. You are his favorite. Don't believe me. Believe His word. It's all in there.

I'm like every one of you. I've struggled (sometimes more than others) with my body image. *Am I tall enough? Am I thin enough? Will I ever like the image staring back in the mirror, or the number on the scale? I wish my thighs looked like hers....*

Let me tell you a little secret. She doesn't like her thighs either.

I reluctantly admit I lived most of my teenage and adult life in a full-blown identity crisis. Until one day, *revelation.* The Holy Spirit began to remind me through his Word who I am:

"God spoke, let us make human beings in our image." ~Genesis 1:27

I am made in the image of the Creator of the universe, God himself! I began to really pay attention to what I said about myself, to myself and to others. If I am made in the image of God and His words are so powerful that the world was created as a result, my words too, are powerful.

I decided that I would no longer allow my emotions to tell me who I am. I decided to talk about what I liked: my strengths, my beauty. When I couldn't come up with anything that day, I decided to let God's Word tell me.

Ephesians 2:10 says that we are his workmanship. Psalms 139 above says I am marvelously made! That means God stepped back and said "Whoa, that's good!" Matthew 10:31 even says that He knows how many hairs are on my head!

My CrossFit gym was a God-send to me. I feel prettiest in the gym. There are no mirrors there or images hanging on the walls reminding me who I'm not. I got off the treadmill (literally) and stopped letting a read-out on a machine tell me if I was successful that day. I learned to engage muscles and become aware of the way my body moves. It gave me a whole new appreciation for how amazing my body is and the work I can accomplish. I decided to change my focus.

So, if his thoughts toward me are good and I am made in His image, I figured I should start appreciating, even celebrating, who I am in Christ. He does!

Dear Heavenly Father, we start by asking that you bind our minds to the mind of Christ. Bind us spirit, soul, and body to the truth of your Word. Please open our hearts to receive what you're saying to us and open our eyes that we may see ourselves like you do. We accept that man looks on the outward appearance, but you, God, look at our hearts. Help us to accept that your ways are higher than ours. We truly desire to live in your presence daily, where we always see things more clearly, and from heaven's perspective. Help us today that we would "let no unwholesome words would come out of our mouths, but only what is useful for building others up, that it may benefit those who listen." (Ephesians 4:29, NIV). Help us to realize that we can defile others even while we speak ill of ourselves. We choose today to speak life over ourselves. We declare, and by an act of our will, accept today that we are fearfully and wonderfully made! In Jesus name we pray, Amen.

WORKOUT 1 — WEEK 4

WARMUP

- [ ] 200-meter jog (0.12 miles)
- [ ] 30 lunges with twist over lunging leg (15 each leg)
- [ ] 30 air squats
- [ ] 10 walk-out/walk-ins
- [ ] 30 jumping jacks
- [ ] 15 jump squats
- [ ] 200-meter run (0.12 miles)

WORKOUT BENCHMARK WORKOUT

"Perfect Fit Benchmark 3" (Record results in your "Workout Log".)

Complete the following as fast as you can with proper form:

- [ ] 100 alternating lunges
- [ ] 100 sit-ups
- [ ] 50 push-ups
- [ ] 50 squats

WORKOUT 2 — WEEK 4

WARMUP

- ☐ 10 walk-out/walk-ins
- ☐ 30 jumping jacks
- ☐ 30 mock kettlebell swings
- ☐ 15 jump squats
- ☐ 5 burpees
- ☐ 400-meter run (0.25 miles)

WORKOUT

10-9-8-7-6-5-4-3-2-1 reps alternating between:

- ☐ Dumbbell push-press
- ☐ Kettlebell swings

AFTERBURN

- ☐ 3 sets of max plank hold with 1 minute rest between each set.[15]

---

15 "Max" simply means that you perform as many reps as you possibly can until you physically can't complete any more. This is also known as "going to failure."

WEEK 5

"And I want women to be modest in their appearance. They should wear decent and appropriate clothing and not draw attention to themselves" ~1 Timothy 2:9, NLT

It goes without saying that our society is chock-full of immodest dressers. Yet sadly, the word "immodest" seems only to be applied in extreme cases of inappropriate exposure. It's increasingly difficult for us as Christian women to maintain modesty when so many fashion magazines, billboards, store windows, and sidewalks propagate styles that are tight, sexy, and provocative.

I never wore belly-bearing shirts as a teenager, but not because I didn't want to; I didn't reveal my stomach because I wasn't confident in my appearance. A few months after I started lifting weights and eating healthily at age sixteen, I was elated to develop and discover muscles I never knew I had: triceps, shoulders, quadriceps, even abs. I remember going to the store and trying on two-piece swimsuits for the first time. I wore them proudly to "boy-girl" swim parties, knowingly rebelling against the Bible's command to be modest so we don't distract others and cause men to stumble into lust.

I've been convicted of my own immodesty even recently. I watched female athletes working out in their sports bras and short shorts, basically fitness lingerie, if you will. They look healthy, strong, *sexy*, and I wanted to look the same. But dressing in this way is dishonoring to God, the men around me, and even my husband.

Looking desirable and sexy is not a bad thing. God created sexual attraction, after all! But when we dress in such a way that draws attention to ourselves and leads men to have impure thoughts (they truly can't help it!), we take what was intended to be a special, sacred gift for one person and tragically demean it, transforming it into an cheap and insignificant way of dress to be seen by anyone who looks our way.

Wearing cute and fashionable clothes that flatter your figure and show accentuate a fit physique is not sinful; I think we all know where to draw the line. But if you find yourself standing in the mirror, scratching your head and asking, *Is this too low? Are these too short?* and on and on, then I'd be willing to bet the piece of clothing in question needs to go back in the closet…or in a trash can.

Though we may be in the world, we are certainly not of it. I pray today that our words, actions, and our wardrobes will reflect who we are in Christ.

"Your beauty should not come from outward adornment, such as braided hair and the wearing of gold jewelry and fine clothes. Instead, it should be that of your inner self, the unfading beauty of a gentle and quiet spirit, which is of great worth in God's sight." ~1 Peter 3:3-4, NIV

Dear Lord, thank You for this day. Thank You for these bodies which You have created fearfully and wonderfully, as David wrote (Psalm 139:14). Thank You for making "all things beautiful in its time," including ourselves (Ecclesiastes 3:11). We pray that we would honor and cherish our beauty by adorning and dressing ourselves in a manner that pleases You and respects our husbands, or future husbands. Help us to be salt and light in the earth so that even in our dress, we can proclaim the Good News of Jesus Christ, Your Son. It's in His Name we pray, Amen.

WORKOUT 1 — WEEK 5

WARMUP

- ☐ 20 lunges each leg
- ☐ 10 high skips (5 each leg)
- ☐ 20 butt-kicks (10 each leg)
- ☐ 20 high-knees (10 each leg)
- ☐ 200-meter (0.12 mile run)
- ☐ 10 air squats
- ☐ 20 arm circles forward
- ☐ 20 arm circles backwards
- ☐ 10 push-ups

WORKOUT BENCHMARK WORKOUT

"Perfect Fit Benchmark 4" (Record results in your "Workout Log".)

Complete the following three rounds as fast as you can with proper form:

- ☐ 800-meter run (0.5 miles)
- ☐ 15 dumbbell thrusters

WORKOUT 2 – WEEK 5

WARMUP

- ☐ 20 reverse lunges (10 each leg)
- ☐ 50 jump rope
- ☐ 20 high-kicks (10 each leg)
- ☐ 10 lateral lunges (5 each leg)
- ☐ 10 walk-out/walk-ins
- ☐ 10 jump squats
- ☐ 20 mountain-climbers (right/left = 1 rep)

WORKOUT

12 minute AMRAP (as many rounds as possible):

- ☐ 12 dips
- ☐ 15 weighted sit-ups (holding dumbbell)
- ☐ 18 lunges (9 each leg)

AFTERBURN

- ☐ 3 sets of max pull-ups with 1 minute rest between sets.[16] (Substitute bent-over dumbbell rows if you don't have a pull-up bar with bands to assist you, or you don't have access to a gym with an assisted pull-up machine.)

---

16 If using an assisted pull-up machine, adjust it to a tough setting at which it's difficult for you to do 10 reps. If you don't have a pull-up bar or assistance, do 3 sets of max dumbbell rows with a heavy pair of dumbbells.

WEEK 6

"Be joyful in hope, patient in affliction, faithful in prayer" ~Romans 12:12, NIV

As both a follower of Jesus and a fitness professional, I've found myself looking to God's Word for guidance, wisdom, strength, and encouragement not only for my spiritual and emotional life, but for my physical life as well. I've found that the verses of the Bible are not one-dimensional, limited to a single context for a one purpose and one purpose only. Quite the opposite! They contain layers upon layers of truth-speaking, life-giving revelation that are just as applicable to our 21st century, high-speed lives as they were to the first Christians who populated the Mediterranean 2,000 years ago.

It may seem strange to some to use a verse such as Romans 12:12 (above) to encourage us in our and fitness journeys, but to me, it's merely another layer to be lifted up and applied to my daily activities.

Most women I know have, or have *had*, some sort of "affliction" regarding their fitness. For some it's weight loss; they simply want to shed a few pound in their midsection or thighs, or tone up before summer arrives. For others, like myself, it's weight gain; a distorted view of our bodies, depression, stress, etc., leaves us tired, weak, and malnourished, and it's time for us to get healthy. Others are battling binge eating disorder or bulimia.

While many people throw in the towel prematurely, those who are "joyful in hope" stick it out, confident that their hard work and discipline will indeed pay off. They feel their clothes fitting more loosely. They see the numbers on the scale getting smaller. They know the weights are getting heavier, pointing directly to their increasing strength. These things testify to their progress. If it weren't for the joy they have, one rooted in the hope of their achieved goals, they could become easily frustrated and discouraged to the point of giving up.

With every spiritual battle we fight, every difficult situation we find ourselves in, the Lord calls us to have hope.

"Yet this I call to mind and therefore I have hope: Because of the Lord's great love we are not consumed, for his compassions never fail. They are new every morning; great is your faithfulness." ~Lamentations 3:21-22, NIV

Have hope that you can reach your goal. You can lose the inches. You can fit into your old jeans. You can run the 5k, lift the weights you want to lift, do a pull-up all by yourself. The Lord cares about your physical fitness even more than you do! Take Jesus' advice and don't worry about tomorrow. Take life one day at a time, hand in hand with Him:

"What I'm trying to do here is to get you to relax, to not be so preoccupied with getting, so you can respond to God's giving. People who don't know God and the way he works fuss over these things, but you know both God and how he works. Steep

your life in God-reality, God-initiative, God-provisions. Don't worry about missing out. You'll find all your everyday human concerns will be met. "* ~Matthew 6:30-33, MSG

Gracious and loving Father, we thank You for your living and active Word. We thank You that You cared so much for us that You not only sent Your Son to die for our sins, but You wrote a love letter to us—our precious Scriptures. We pray that the verses we read will take root in our hearts, energizing and empowering us to live victoriously for You, hoping in You, trusting in You in all things. No matter what we're up against in life, from relationship struggles to weight loss battles, we know that You care more than anyone that we come out conquerors! We ask You to give us the strength to call upon You when we grow weak and discouraged. Help us to keep our eyes on the prize, not the problem. In Your Son Jesus' Name we pray, Amen.

WORKOUT 1 — WEEK 6

WARMUP

2 rounds:

- ☐ 20 butt-kicks (10 each leg)
- ☐ 20 high-knees (1o each leg)
- ☐ 20 mountain-climbers (right/left = 1 rep)
- ☐ 15 air squats
- ☐ 15 push-ups
- ☐ 5 burpees

WORKOUT

Complete the following as fast as you can with proper form:

18 rounds:

- ☐ 10 jump rope
- ☐ 3 strict dumbbell presses
- ☐ 4 box jumps (20-inch box)

WORKOUT 2 — WEEK 6

WARMUP

3 rounds:

- [ ] 20 reverse lunges (10 each leg)
- [ ] 5 walk-outs
- [ ] 10 air squats
- [ ] 10 push-ups

WORKOUT

Complete, with proper form:

15-12-9-6-3 reps of:

- [ ] Sumo deadlift high-pulls with kettlebell
- [ ] Oblique twists holding kettlebell (each side is one rep)
- [ ] Jump squats

AFTERBURN

- [ ] 3 sets of max pushups with 1 minute rest between sets.

WEEK 7

By   Anna Kugel

Age   23

Occupation Elementary school teacher

"God will make this happen, for he who calls you is faithful" ~1 Thessalonians 5:24, NLT

"Know therefore that the LORD your God is God; he is the faithful God, keeping his covenant of love to a thousand generations of those who love him and keep his commands." ~Deuteronomy 7:9, NLT

The best months of my life were those that included a good and trusted friend to keep me accountable, healthy but yummy food options, and a disciplined daily routine. During the last semester of my junior year of college my friend Allison and I determined to keep each other accountable to get up every morning before class—even if that meant literally rolling out of bed—and going together to work out.

I never felt more strengthened in every way than I have that semester. I was able to keep a disciplined routine starting the first thing of each day because I had a solid and trusting relationship to keep me at it. But a strong, sustainable determination to be fit and healthy must come first from a personal relationship with Jesus Christ. If He was not first in my life, strengthening me to keep pursuing these vital priorities, I would have had no desire to even have a trusted accountability partner in Allison.

It all starts with knowing Christ on a personal level and by surrounding yourself with His Word and other people who believe what Scripture says as well. Once this is in place, He will readily put healthy desires in your mind and heart. Then it is our responsibility to take action and find ways to make these desires happen.

I challenge you to make time to work out several days this week. It takes some consideration to figure out when workouts will "work out" in your schedule, but God will give you wisdom. Before anything else, sit with Your Savior. Ask Him to guide your week one day at a time and make His desires your desires.

Lord Jesus, I pray you would keep fanning the flame within my spirit, helping me to continue a life that is fully pleasing to you, from my time working out to my time on my knees before you. As I meet with you and you place your desires in my heart, continue your work in me until its completion. Thank you in advance for what you will do and for the blessings time spent devoted to you will bring. Amen.

WORKOUT 1 — WEEK 7

WARMUP

- [ ] 20 reverse lunges (10 each leg)
- [ ] 50 jump rope
- [ ] 10 lateral lunges (5 each leg)
- [ ] 10 walk-out/walk-ins
- [ ] 10 jump squats
- [ ] 20 mountain-climbers (right/left = 1 rep)

WORKOUT

Complete the following as fast as you can, maintaining proper form:

3 minute AMREP:[17]

- [ ] 400-meter run (0.25 miles)
- [ ] Max push-ups
- [ ] *Rest* 1 minute.

4 minute AMREP:

- [ ] 400-meter run
- [ ] Max pull-ups (sub bent-over dumbbell rows if you don't have access to a pull-up bar or assisted pull-up machine)
- [ ] *Rest* 1 minute.

5 minute AMREP:

- [ ] 400-meter run
- [ ] Max burpees

---

17 "AMREP," not to be confused with "AMRAP," stands for "As Many REPS as Possible." Count how many reps you do of the given exercise.

WORKOUT 2 — WEEK 7

WARMUP

- ☐ 20 lunges each leg
- ☐ 10 high skips (5 each leg)
- ☐ 20 butt-kicks (10 each leg)
- ☐ 20 high-knees (10 each leg)
- ☐ 200-meter (0.12 mile run)
- ☐ 10 air squats
- ☐ 20 arm circles forward
- ☐ 20 arm circles backwards
- ☐ 10 push-ups

WORKOUT

Complete the following as fast as you can, maintaining proper form:

5 rounds:

- ☐ 20 dumbbell squats
- ☐ 15 reverse lunges each leg
- ☐ 10 kettlebell swings

WEEK 8

By	Colby Satterfield
Age	28
Occupation	Engineering Technician and Aspiring CrossFit Competitive Athlete and Motivator

"But those who hope in the Lord will renew their strength. They will soar on wings like eagles; they will run and not grow weary, they will walk and not be faint" -Isaiah 40:31, NIV

I remember reading this scripture over and over during times of despair just a few months back. Every day I would read it and feel its power. I'd even feel stronger even *physically*. I emphasize the word "physically" because at this time I wasn't fully embracing the Lord. To be honest I was scared.

How many times have you walked up to a loaded barbell and let it defeat you before even picking it up? It's because you didn't commit to it. You weren't confident, and you let fear overtake you.

We've all felt this feeling of fear and frustration in some fashion or another, and it makes for a useful metaphor describing our relationship with God at times. You see, it is only when we fully commit ourselves to living for God that we believe and KNOW that we can do anything through him.

I had thrown myself into a regimen of train, train, and train in order not to deal with my emotional state. Sure I was lifting more, but I felt heavier than ever. Not weight-wise, but in my soul. I hadn't asked the Lord to help heal my spirit, and my gym family needed that spirit and heart as I needed theirs. One night I fell on my knees and proclaimed that I couldn't go on this way, that I was more alone than ever. Meanwhile, the Lord had already placed a support group right in front of me. He said: "They are strong with me. Embrace them."

I knew without a doubt that He was speaking about my gym community. The minute I walked through those doors, He'd already been at work preparing me for the future, surrounding me with strong Christians who loved the Lord were going to ignite that hunger in me to learn more, to live for others not myself.

There it is: COMMUNITY. The box has been a place to build a strong foundation in Him. It humbles me and teaches me the patience and consistency that I, and I think all of us, need every day. I tell you all of this to encourage you to go the Lord, embrace your fitness family or whoever it is you work out with, and build each up each other in Him. Keep fighting for your goals because God is fighting for you. Do this and watch the PR's (code for "Personal Records") start racking up in life and in the box.

"Because you have so little faith. I tell you the truth, if you have faith as small as a mustard seed, you can say to this mountain, 'Move from here to there' and it will move. Nothing will be impossible for you." ~Matthew 17:20, NIV

Dear Lord, we ask for Your presence to be strong every day and in everything we do, that You would keep us focused on You in our hearts, souls and minds as You have commanded us. We thank You for the strong Christian women that You have placed in our lives and ask that You would use us to encourage others who also need encouragement, need refreshing, need YOU, Lord. In Jesus Christ's name, who gave His sinless life for us, Amen.

WORKOUT 1 — WEEK 8

WARMUP

3 rounds:

- ☐ 10 reverse lunges (5 each leg)
- ☐ 10 high skips (5 each leg)
- ☐ 20 high-kicks (10 each leg)
- ☐ 10 wall squats
- ☐ 15 mock kettlebell swings

WORKOUT

8 minute AMRAP:

- ☐ 10 double-unders (if unable to do double-unders, perform 30 regular single jump rope)
- ☐ 10 suitcase deadlifts
- ☐ 3 burpees

AFTERBURN

- ☐ 50 superman

WORKOUT 2 — WEEK 8

WARMUP

- [ ] 200-meter jog (0.12 miles)
- [ ] 30 lunges with twist over lunging leg (15 each leg)
- [ ] 30 air squats
- [ ] 10 walk-out/walk-ins
- [ ] 30 jumping jacks
- [ ] 15 jump squats
- [ ] 200-meter run (0.12 miles)

WORKOUT

Complete the following as fast as you can with proper form:

- [ ] 400-meter run (0.25 miles)
- [ ] 30-20-10 reps alternating:
- [ ] Dumbbell push-press
- [ ] Weighted sit-ups (holding dumbbell)
- [ ] 400-meter run

WEEK 9

"...and we take captive every thought to make it obedient to Christ"
~2 Corinthians 10:5, MSG

Holding my tongue is something I've been trained to do from a very early age. Commenting to my daycare teacher that she remarkably resembled the Wicked Witch of the West was not nice. I shouldn't have said something like that, even if I was at the outspoken, unbridled age of three and a half.

One of my favorite Disney cartoons growing up was *Bambi*. We all know the famous line spoken by Bambi's energetic bunny-friend, Thumper: *"If you can't say something nice, don't say nothin' at all."*

I assume that most all of us had parents and grandparents who, since we were knee-high to a pig's eye, have been using this rabbit's wisdom to teach us politeness. What I have *not* been so adept at is holding my thoughts...

King Solomon instructed us to guard our hearts because they are wellsprings of life (Proverbs 4:23). Over nine-hundred years later, Jesus said that we speak from the overflow of our hearts (Matthew 12:34). If our hearts are full of hope and joy, we will speak optimistically and scatter the storm clouds of worry and fear that the enemy so often sends into our skies. But while keeping our tongues in check is vital to a victorious life, so too is maintaining a mind filled with godly thoughts that build up and encourage, not tear down and dishearten.

In her book *Battlefield of the Mind: Winning the Battle in Your Mind*, evangelist and author Joyce Meyer writes that we cannot have a positive life and a negative mind simultaneously. Isn't that so true? If we think negatively about ourselves, we can't help but be in low spirits, and to quote Solomon again, "a crushed spirit, who can bear?" (Proverbs 18:14). Pessimistic, worrisome, fearful, and self-pitying thoughts translate into a miserable and depressed life, one that Jesus came to save us from (John 10:10). And we can only keep the Happy Camper act up for so long before our smile muscles cave to the pulling forces of insincerity and weariness, and we have a meltdown.

Philippians 4:8 encourages us to think on what is true, noble, right, pure, lovely, admirable, and praiseworthy. When you start feeling discouraged, replace what *isn't* going right with what *is*. Think of all that God has done for you, and think on His promises to prosper and bless you, and that He—this very moment—is working all things together for your good (Jeremiah 29:11, Romans 8:28). Remember that we are daily at war with Satan and his invisible armies whose mission it is to derail you from your purpose on this planet and plunder your joy in the process. The Word of God is the most powerful weapon we have against their attacks. Let's use it! Let's fill our minds with it daily and commit to memory verses that we can easily pull out like a light saber to extinguish the darts of the devil.

"Your Word is a lamp unto my feet and a light unto my path." ~Psalm 119:105, ESV

Almighty God, we thank you for the precious gift of your Word and its hope-filled, life-giving, lie-destroying power. We thank You for all the wonderful plans You have for us and that none of us are without hope, nor deserving of condemnation. Your Son has saved us from the curse of sin, and we are heirs in Your eternal kingdom! Help us to live like the royal priesthood we are—joyfully and triumphantly, and full of hope and light for a world desperate for your love and grace. We pray this in Jesus' name, Amen.

WORKOUT 1 — WEEK 9

WARMUP

3 rounds:

- [ ] 200-meter jog (0.12 miles)
- [ ] 30 air squats
- [ ] 5 walk-outs
- [ ] 10 high skips (5 each leg)
- [ ] 20 butt-kicks (10 each leg)
- [ ] 20 high-knees (10 each leg)
- [ ] 5 burpees

WORKOUT

Complete the following as fast as you can with proper form:

21-15-9 reps of:

- [ ] Dumbbell squats
- [ ] Alternating dumbbell lunges
- [ ] Double-unders (sub 63-45-27 single jump ropes if unable to do double-unders)

AFTERBURN

- [ ] Tabata push-ups[18]

---

18 "Tabata," named for Japanese scientist Izumi Tabata who developed it, is the name of a type of training in which you perform a specified activity for twenty seconds and then rest for ten seconds. You repeat this sequence eight times for a total of four minutes.

WORKOUT 2 — WEEK 9

WARMUP

- [ ] 20 lunges (10 each leg)
- [ ] 10 walk-out/walk-ins
- [ ] 20 scorpions (10 each side)
- [ ] 20 reverse lunges (10 each leg)
- [ ] 50 jump rope
- [ ] 10 burpees

WORKOUT

- [ ] 20 minute AMRAP
- [ ] 400-meter run (0.25 miles)
- [ ] 15 box jumps (sub broad jumps if you don't have a plyo box)
- [ ] 20 sit-ups

WEEK 18

"The tongue has the power of life and death, and those who love it will eat its fruit." ~Proverbs 18:21, NIV

"I'll always have this flab."

"I'll never be able to fit into my old jeans."

"I'll never be able to lift that much weight."

"I don't have enough self-control to maintain a healthy diet."

"I wish I could be disciplined enough to work out consistently, but I don't have it in me."

According to the Solomon, the wisest man who ever lived, that's all toxic language! (1 Kings 4:30) Sadly, I don't think most people realize just how potent their words really are. The very first chapter of the Bible demonstrates the power of words by showing us how the universe reacts and obeys God's commands:

"And God said, 'Let there be light,' and there was light" ~Genesis 1:3, NIV.

Had God said, "Let there be eternal darkness and unparalleled chaos," you can bet we'd be miserably moping about like moles, stuck inside a bleak, dystopian nightmare. But because our God is good and the immutable embodiment of Love itself, we enjoy the dawn of the rising sun and marvel at the matchless colors of dusk (1 John 4:8, NIV).

I believe the Holy Spirit inspired Moses, the writer of Genesis, to describe creation the way he did so an example could be set of how we're to use our tongues, as well as illustrate the perceptible effects our speech has on our lives. When we say negative things about ourselves, we are speaking a metaphorical universe of darkness into existence. Continuing to comment on how displeased we are with our bodies or how much we wish we looked like somebody else only fills us with self-pity and discouragement, making it all the more difficult, if not impossible, to trust that God can guide us to our goals...and beyond them...

*"Now to him who is able to do **immeasurably more** than all we ask or imagine, according to his power that is at work within us, to him be glory in the church and in Christ Jesus..."* -Ephesians 3:20-21 (emphasis added)

Remember that that mighty muscle inside your mouth is meant for more than enjoying food with your taste buds and enjoying conversations with your best buds; it's for speaking *life*! When mountains materialize in your path, don't shudder at its size and state how scary it is. Instead, remember and obey the words of Jesus and tell that mountain to move! (Mark 11:23). No matter if the mountain is a major life transition looming on the horizon or a reflection in your mirror, you have the power of the Holy Spirit inside you to help you chase it into the sea.

Lord of light and love, we praise You for showing us how wonderful words can be and for also warning us against their ability to tear down and destroy. We ask you to forgive us for speaking recklessly and impulsively at times, and pray that Your soul-soothing Scriptures would enter our minds and ignite our tongues with life. Thank You for sending the Living Word, Your Son Jesus, to forgive us of all our sins and teach us how to live healthy, fruitful, victorious lives. In His Name, Amen.

WORKOUT 1 — WEEK 18

WARMUP

- [ ] 400-meter jog
- [ ] 10 walk-outs
- [ ] 20 arm circles forward
- [ ] 20 arm circles reverse
- [ ] 20 mountain-climbers (right/left is 1 rep)
- [ ] 20 air squats
- [ ] 10 burpees

WORKOUT

Complete the following as fast as you can with proper form:

4 rounds:

- [ ] 18 dumbbell thrusters
- [ ] 14 dumbbell oblique twists (each side is one rep)
- [ ] 10 bent-over dumbbell rows

WORKOUT 2 — WEEK 10

WARMUP

2 rounds:

- [ ] 20 reverse lunges (10 each leg)
- [ ] 15 air squats
- [ ] 20 lunges with oblique twist (10 each leg)
- [ ] 10 high skips (5 each side)
- [ ] 10 scorpions (5 each side)

WORKOUT

9 minute AMRAP:

- [ ] 10 dips
- [ ] 10 suitcase deadlifts
- [ ] 100-meter run (0.06 miles)

AFTERBURN

- [ ] Tabata lunges (either stationary or walking)

WEEK 11

By   Heidi Luong
Age   35
Occupation Mom of two and CrossFit Coach

"Be strong in the Lord and in His mighty power. Put on all of God's armor so that you will be able to stand firm against all strategies of the devil" ~Ephesians 6:10-11, NLT

What is my vision, plan, or dream? What do I pursue? And what am I fighting for?

Whether it's happiness, health and fitness, a joyful marriage, being the world's best mom, a good sister, friend, daughter or employee, or even attaining goals like going for that next PR, we daily find ourselves doing and achieving what matters most to us. We as women love to make lists and place check marks beside accomplished tasks. But sometimes we get in the way of ourselves. We become overly focused on tasks at-hand and soon forget or push aside the things that can, well...*wait.*

Satan is a deceiver and his number one goal is to steal, kill, and destroy (John 10:10). And his target is us! We have a real-life battle to fight every day as war is being waged for our souls and for eternity. We can have the best intentions in the world and not ever really accomplish anything of true value. Knowing this, the enemy does all he can to distract, confuse, and attack our hearts when we are not on guard. But there is Good News...

We have a loving everlasting, eternal Father in Heaven who has given His Son to die for our sins. Praise God! He has also given us his Holy Spirit and the sword of his Word to wield at the attacks of Satan in our lives each day. To be guarded and aware we have to be eternally-minded and focused. To be prepared must be in the Word of Truth everyday! This is our armor and our source of true strength. I've heard the saying "strong is the new skinny" but in reality, strong is a way of life, as it should be for us, a day-in and day-out receiving of his best for us.

The Bible tells us of the blessings of coming to Him daily. In hardships and struggles, we are able to abide in him and persevere with a promise and a future hope, for His yoke is easy and His burden is light (Matt 11:30). In our weak moments of growth, humility, service to others, and throwing all our boasts and crowns at His feet, Jesus Christ is glorified. He will carry us through our struggles and daily battles. However, to receive this kind of blessing and promise we have to "walk circumspectly, not as fools, but as wise, redeeming the time, for the days are evil" (Ephesians 5:15-16).

In my gym, I see the model of "disciple", the casting off of all worry and doubt and just doing the work and persevering toward goals one day at a time. Little by little, through hardships, frustrations and lots of sore muscles, I see improvements made and efforts achieved. I encourage and motivate my friends to press on or watch out for obstacles that hinder. The community is a caring one and that is a beautiful reminder of living outside of myself and living within God's love and care. The Lord has called me to become a coach so that I might reach others where they are, relate, and help them on their journey as I am growing in mine. My aim is to do all of this to the glory of God (1 Corinthians10:31).

Dear Lord, I lift your name on high! You are the giver of life and the Author and Finisher of all our days. In our weaknesses you are strong and in our battles you are mighty to save and overcome. Thank you so much for the community found inside the gym, or wherever we train, and the things you are teaching us. Lord, my prayer is this: "therefore we also, since we are surrounded by so great a cloud of witnesses, let us lay aside every weight, and the sin which so easily ensnares us, and let us run with endurance the race that is set before us, looking unto Jesus, the author and finisher of our faith, who for the joy that was set before Him endured the cross, despising the shame, and has sat down at the right hand of the throne of God (Hebrews 12:1-2). I pray for strength and encouragement to help us be eternally-minded with thoughts set upon our prize where rust and moth and death cannot destroy. We are more than conquerors in Christ! Lord, Our victory is in You! In your Son Jesus' name we pray, Amen.

WORKOUT 1 — WEEK 11

WARMUP

- ☐ 200-meter run
- ☐ 20 high-kicks (10 each leg)
- ☐ 20 air squats
- ☐ 30 lunges with oblique twist (15 each side)
- ☐ 10 squat jumps
- ☐ 30 mock kettlebell swings
- ☐ 10 push-ups

WORKOUT

Complete the following as fast as you can with proper form:

21-18-15-12-9-6-3 reps of:

- ☐ Kettlebell swings
- ☐ Burpees

WORKOUT 2 — WEEK 11

WARMUP

3 rounds:

- [ ] 10 high-skips (5 each side)
- [ ] 20 butt-kicks (20 each side)
- [ ] 20 high-knees (20 each side)
- [ ] 100 meter run (0.06 miles)
- [ ] 20 scorpions (10 each side)
- [ ] 10 jump squats

WORKOUT

12 minute AMRAP:

- [ ] 200-meter run
- [ ] 20 reverse lunges (10 each leg)
- [ ] 15 goblet squats (holding kettlebell)

AFTERBURN

- [ ] 100 sit-ups for time

WEEK 12

"Come near to God and he will come near to you." ~James 4:8, NIV

What is it that's troubling you, worrying you, discouraging you today? Have you talked about it with the Lord?

There was a time not too many years ago when I only let God handle the "big things" in my life, i.e., family, friends, relationships, school. The issues I categorized as "minor," like my unhealthy obsession with exercise and self-destructive fixation on maintaining a double-digit scale reading, I didn't even consider praying for. Though I recognized, by a host of alarming symptoms, that I was in a real physical battle, part of me didn't believe God could really help me. But the moment I hit rock bottom and called out to God in abject desperation, worry, and fear, I felt the unseen arms of the Father lifting me out of the mire. He'd been there watching, waiting, yearning for me to surrender my burdens to Him the whole time.

Yes the Lord is the sole possessor of many magnificent and unfathomable titles, like "King of Kings," "Majesty on High," and "Consuming Fire," but He also has names that bid us come and discover peace and find solutions to every struggle in life, names like "Breath of Life," "Deliverer," "Comforter," and "Good Shepherd" (1 Timothy 6:15, Hebrews 1:3, Deuteronomy 4:24, Revelation 11:11, Romans 11:26, Isaiah 55:4, John 10:11).

Paul writes in Romans that because we are God's children, we may call out to Him: "*Abba*, Father" (Romans 8:15). If your dad is anything like mine was, he can be a stern disciplinarian when he needs to be, but whenever you experience pain, whether physical or emotional, he's there to scoop you up and doctor your wounds with the wisdom and TLC only daddies can provide. If our dads can be this loving, how much more wonderful is our Heavenly Father when we run to Him? (Luke 11:13).

Our Good Shepherd, we praise you for being our loving Abba, our heavenly Daddy who inclines His ear to hear our every concern, handle all of our cares, and replace our fears, longings, angst, and unrest with the fruits of your Spirit, fruits like joy, peace, patience, and faithfulness. We pray for the faith to trust You with all things, Father. In the Name of Your Son Jesus we pray, Amen.

WORKOUT 1 — WEEK 12

WARMUP

- [ ] 20 lunges (10 each leg)
- [ ] 10 walk-out/walk-ins
- [ ] 20 scorpions (10 each side)
- [ ] 20 reverse lunges (10 each leg)
- [ ] 50 jump rope
- [ ] 10 burpees

WORKOUT

14 minute AMRAP:

- [ ] 30 jump rope
- [ ] 20 sit-ups
- [ ] 10 pull-ups (sub bent-over dumbbell rows if you don't have a pull-up bar)

WORKOUT 2 — WEEK 12

WARMUP

- ☐ 20 lunges (10 each leg)
- ☐ 10 walk-out/walk-ins
- ☐ 20 scorpions (10 each side)
- ☐ 20 reverse lunges (10 each leg)
- ☐ 50 jump rope
- ☐ 10 burpees

WORKOUT

Complete the following as fast as you can, maintaining proper form:

- ☐ 800-meter run (0.5 miles)
- ☐ 20 push-ups
- ☐ 400-meter run (0.25 miles)
- ☐ 40 push-ups
- ☐ 200-meter run (0.12 miles)
- ☐ 60 push-ups

AFTERBURN

- ☐ 50 kettlebell swings for time

WEEK 13

By   Rebecca White

Age   36

Occupation Salon owner and hairstylist

"So here's what I want you to do, God helping you: Give your bodies as a living sacrifice to God- Take your everyday, ordinary life—your sleeping, eating, going-to-work, and walking-around life—and place it before God as an offering. Embracing what God does for you is the best thing you can do for him. Don't become so well-adjusted to your culture that you fit into it without even thinking. Instead, fix your attention on God. You'll be changed from the inside out. Readily recognize what he wants from you, and quickly respond to it. Unlike the culture around you, always dragging you down to its level of immaturity, God brings the best out of you, develops well-formed maturity in you" -Roman 12:1-2, MSG

How can one do this? How can one give her whole self to a God she cannot see? On a woman's wedding night, it feels a bit awkward to give her body to this man she's never been with intimately before. Yes, it's exciting, and there's been much anticipation leading up to their first night honeymooning together, but there's also an unavoidable feeling of vulnerability as she gives all of herself to another person, knowing there's no turning back. How much harder it is sometimes to give our bodies, our lives, to God, whom we've never even seen. All we have is faith that our decision to follow and trust Him is the best we'll ever make.

I've learned that developing a real, meaningful relationship with God means spending a great amount of time in His Word. There are numerous ways in this Information Age that make that a simple goal to achieve. Free podcasts, television shows, and talk radio allow a busy life the opportunity to plug in to God's Word while on the go.

The Bible says that believing comes by hearing the Word of God (Romans 10:17). The more time we spend seeking God through His Word, the greater our faith will grow to be. We will learn He is trustworthy, that He loves us, that we are his prized possession, His beautiful, beloved bride. We can learn to be intimate and vulnerable with Him; He no longer feels like a stranger, but conversely, a Perfect Friend, a Doting Daddy, a Loving Husband.

I want to know my true value, I want to have the best brought out in me. I want maturity that comes from the number of hours I spend in God's Word, not the number of years I've lived on this earth. The more I seek God, the more I find Him, and all of these things and much more are added to me. My value increases. My capacity to love and be loved increases. All of the desires of my heart are filled, and I am whole, I am safe. I am in the arms of a man that will never fail me, never leave me, never use me. I am held.

Daddy God, we want more of You. More comprehension, more understanding of who You are and of who we are in You. Wrap my thoughts in humility around You. Give me the mind of Christ so that we will have the ability to see with eyes of love and understanding, even through the toughest moments. We need Your transforming power to heal what is broken inside of us, to strengthen what is weak, and to equip us for Your kingdom purposes while we inhabit these fleshly bodies on earth. We devote ourselves to Your Word. Pull us in deeper. Take our hands and help us trust You to guide us into the unknown, walking by faith, not by sight, out of darkness, into Your marvelous Light. Amen.

WORKOUT 1 — WEEK 13

WARMUP

- [ ] 400-meter jog
- [ ] 10 walk-outs
- [ ] 20 high-kicks (10 each leg)
- [ ] 20 arm circles forward
- [ ] 20 arm circles reverse
- [ ] 20 mountain-climbers (right/left is 1 rep)
- [ ] 20 air squats
- [ ] 10 burpees

WORKOUT

6 minute AMRAP:

- [ ] 5 pull-ups (Substitute bent-over dumbbell rows if you don't have a pull-up bar with bands to assist you, or you don't have access to a gym with an assisted pull-up machine.)
- [ ] 15 squats
- [ ] *Rest* 2 minutes.

6 minute AMRAP:

- [ ] 8 push-ups
- [ ] 10 suitcase deadlifts

WORKOUT 2 — WEEK 13

WARMUP

2 rounds:

- [ ] 20 reverse lunges (10 each leg)
- [ ] 15 air squats
- [ ] 20 lunges with oblique twist (10 each leg)
- [ ] 10 high skips (5 each side)
- [ ] 10 scorpions (5 each side)

WORKOUT

Complete the following as fast as you can, maintaining proper form:

10 rounds:

- [ ] 5 box jumps
- [ ] 200-meter run

AFTERBURN

- [ ] Tabata superman

WEEK 14

"And do not forget to do good and to share with others, for with such sacrifices God is pleased" ~Hebrews 13:16, NIV

I don't know about you, but in my life, "doing good," as this verse instructs, isn't too hard to forget. For example, just this week I was entering the grocery store when I spotted an elderly woman having a difficult time pulling a shopping cart out of its row. I didn't think twice about going over and yanking it free for her. And when it was apparent that a family at the airport recently was running late for their flight, I remembered to "do good" and insist they pass in front of me in the security line. My mama didn't raise no ill-mannered fool!

What doesn't come so easily to me is the "to share" part of to-day's Scripture. In each of the occurrences above, I hardly spoke. A shy and introverted person by nature, I'm not one to strike up con-versation with distressed grandmothers at the store or stressed-out families on-the-go. I'm not one who likes to share with strangers.

But sharing is a major calling and responsibility for us as Christians. How else is the Gospel and God's love made known to the world but through sharing? How else do we let others know how Christ has saved, set free, and transformed us but through opening our mouths, pulling out our pens, or firing up our computers to reach hurting, wandering souls? It is only when we exit our cozy turtle shells, forget restrictive adjectives and labels like "timid," "introverted" and "loner," and allow the Holy Spirit to direct our steps and inspire our words that God's Kingdom work can be accomplished through us.

Now, I'm not saying that we must quote John 3:16 to every cashier, courtesy clerk, and cab driver we encounter; however, based on God's Word, we must not be opposed to or intimidated by such opportunities. If you feel God directing you to dialogue with someone whose day needs brightening, whose hope needs stirring, whose heart needs softening, trust that the Lord will give you the words to say and bring to your remembrance the things his Son has told you in Scripture (John 14:26).

No matter how uncomfortable it may make us to ask a stranger if we can pray for them or to invite a mere acquaintance to church, we must remember that it is Christ in us who is truly doing the work. He is the one knocking at the heart's door of those we share him with. We should be glad and grateful to announce his visit, knowing that the sacrifice of our time and the escape from our comfort zones pleases our Lord and Savior.

Father in Heaven, we thank you for the abundant encouragement and exhortation we find in your word. Thank you for the Bible, your love letter to us, and the treasure trove of tremendous truths and powerful promises it contains. Even the meekest and most shy among us are moved to action and interaction with others by verses like today's which tell us that sacrificing to share and do good bring you delight. Place on our hearts those individuals we are to talk with and pray for. Drop onto our tongues the perfect words to say. And provide us with the humbleness and boldness to do this without inhibition or self-consciousness. We know we can do all things through your Son, in whose ever-loving, ever-encouraging, everlasting name we pray, Amen.

WORKOUT 1 — WEEK 14

WARMUP

- ☐ 200-meter run
- ☐ 30 air squats
- ☐ 30 lunges with oblique twist (15 each side)
- ☐ 10 squat jumps
- ☐ 30 mock kettlebell swings
- ☐ 10 push-ups

WORKOUT

18 minute AMRAP:

- ☐ 15 kettlebell swings
- ☐ 15 air squats
- ☐ 20 mountain-climbers (right/left is 1 rep)

WORKOUT 2 — WEEK 14

WARMUP

3 rounds:

- [ ] 20 reverse lunges (10 each leg)
- [ ] 5 walk-outs
- [ ] 10 air squats
- [ ] 10 push-ups

WORKOUT

- [ ] Tabata reverse lunges
- [ ] *Rest* 2 minutes
- [ ] Tabata sit-ups
- [ ] *Rest* 2 minutes
- [ ] Tabata forward lunges

AFTERBURN

- [ ] 5 100-meter sprints, resting ninety seconds between sprints

WEEK 15

By   Rachel Verme
Age   31
Occupation Nurse and Stay-at-home Mom

"Let go [of your concerns]! Then you will know that I am God. I rule the nations. I rule the earth." ~Psalms 46:10, God's Word Translation

For most of my life, I have doubted who I am in Christ. I have had the thought that God must have made a mistake in putting me together. I am naturally introverted, have struggled with my self-esteem and self-worth, and hated parts of my personality. For years, I constantly compared myself to others who were outgoing, popular, etc. Add to my constant insecurities the extra college and baby weight of my 20's, I was a wreck.

I hated looking in the mirror. I hated my husband looking at me. I hated going to the gym and wearing shorts. I hated what I had become. I was very athletic in high school and had a track scholarship for college, but even then I doubted that at 120 pounds and a size 4 I was good enough.

After my first baby, my dad (whom I love and adore) made a comment one day when I had just finished "working out" at a gym (I don't think I broke a sweat that day on the elliptical). He stated in a very personal and gut-ripping way that I needed to take better care of myself, if not for me, but for my husband, while referencing my "pooch." This stung straight to my heart, as you can imagine.

I went home and cried in the shower and for the first time in 29 years and to pray about my struggles with my weight and eating. I gave it to God, and as the shower washed my tears away, I felt refreshed. I got out of the shower and spent the next hour journaling what God was showing me...

"I am fearfully and wonderfully made" (Psalm 139:14). He knew what he was doing when he made me. He made me this way on purpose, knowing that I would need to seek him for help constantly with my issues with weight, diet, and self-control as a way to fully rely on Him. It was still a couple years later (another pregnancy and baby to nurse got in the way) before I started to really put my workouts and dieting into God's hands and not my own.

I started running and then found a group of girls that pushed me to run farther than two to three miles. They started encouraging me into longer distances. We raced together, prayed together, and they pushed me every step of the way. Then a friend started talking about her CrossFit gym, and I was curious. My friend told me the workouts were only ten to twenty minutes long, but high-intensity, guaranteed to get you fit and toned.

I decided to give her gym a try, not quite sure I would like it. I was hooked after the first week! I was sore, loved the challenges, and thrived on the encouragement from the coaches. I now look forward to my workouts, and can't wait till I can RX more of them.[19] I love the accountability of my run group and the motivation and inspiration of my CrossFit gym.

During the last year, one of the other key lessons I've learned is to take every thought captive and "let no unwholesome word come out of my mouth" when my mind wants to dwell on negative and derogatory thoughts about myself (2 Corinthians 10:5, Ephesians 4:29). I would never tell someone else they're fat, ugly, or no good, so why did I think it was okay to say it about myself? When I think these thoughts, I am saying that God made a mistake with me.

Do I still slip up on my eating habits, slack off on workouts, or compare myself to the girl next to me and talk down on myself? Of course. I am human. God uses these moments of weakness to remind me that I need him every step of the way. So even though I had a handful of Rolo's and a bag of chips at work today, I am still his beloved creation and worthy of his grace, mercy, and unfailing love.

19 "RX" means doing the workout as prescribed by the coaches. "Going RX" means you didn't have to scale by using lighter weights, the help of a resistance band, etc.

Lord, you, the Creator of the world, Author of Life, made me. You planned me before time began. You know my struggles, you know me intimately. I praise you that you know what you are doing with me and through me. I submit my workouts, my dieting, my health, all to you. Forgive me when I doubt myself, talk down on myself, or stop trying. Continue to place people in my life that I need for accountability, encouragement, and instruction. Make me aware of who I am encouraging or motivating because of what you are doing in my life. Help me to claim your word for strength. Remind me when I am slipping from my goals. Help me not turn my back on your love and power that you have for me. In Jesus' name, Amen.

WORKOUT 1 — WEEK 15

WARMUP

2 rounds:

- [ ] 20 stationary lunges (10 each leg)
- [ ] 20 stationary butt-kicks (10 each leg)
- [ ] 20 stationary high-knees (10 each leg)
- [ ] 15 air squats
- [ ] 10 push-ups
- [ ] 5 burpees

WORKOUT BENCHMARK WORKOUT

"Perfect Fit Benchmark 1" (Record results in your "Workout Log") and compare your results with Week 1, Workout 1!

16 minute AMRAP (as many rounds as possible):

- [ ] 5 pull-ups (Substitute bent-over dumbbell rows if you don't have a pull-up bar with bands to assist you, or you don't have access to a gym with an assisted pull-up machine.)
- [ ] 7 push-ups
- [ ] 9 air squats

WORKOUT 2 — WEEK 15

WARMUP

- [ ] 400-meter jog
- [ ] 10 walk-outs
- [ ] 20 arm circles forward
- [ ] 20 arm circles reverse
- [ ] 20 mountain-climbers (right/left is 1 rep)
- [ ] 20 air squats
- [ ] 5 jump squats

WORKOUT

Complete the following as fast as you can, maintaining proper form:

- [ ] 100-meter run (0.06 miles)
- [ ] 20 burpees
- [ ] 5 dumbbell thrusters
- [ ] 200-meter run (0.12 miles)
- [ ] 15 burpees
- [ ] 10 dumbbell thrusters
- [ ] 400-meter run (0.25 miles)
- [ ] 25 burpees
- [ ] 15 dumbbell thrusters

WEEK 16

"Therefore there is now no condemnation for those who are in Christ Jesus" ~Romans 8:1, NASB

Not long ago, a Christian fitness model shared news on Facebook that grieved my heart. Her new husband, a Christian musician, had been uninvited from performing at several churches because of explicit and provocative photographs his wife had appeared in early on in her modeling career.

Heartbroken, this beautiful, Jesus-loving young woman posted a video in which she emotionally voiced her regrets for having posed in sexy, skimpy bikinis and workout attire. She cautioned aspiring models against beginning their careers in a similar fashion, underscoring the importance of self-respect, staying true to one's values, and also guarding the hearts and minds of men who are more prone to lust by simply looking at a picture.

Years back, she was convicted by the Holy Spirit and stopped displaying her fit physique in this immodest, worldly way. Now, however, the mistakes of her past are still being condemned by others, even by brothers and sisters within the Church.

The New Testament states over and over again that we are no longer condemned for our sins, past, present, or future. Nor will we receive the punishment we deserve. We have been justified— Christ's blood paid for it all! (Romans 8:31-39, John, 3:17, 18, John 5:24).

One of my favorite examples of Christ's extravagant grace and tenderness is found in John chapter eight. A woman has been caught in the act of adultery, the penalty for which is death by stoning. Jesus said to her accusers:

"'Let any one of you who is without sin be the first to throw a stone at her.' Again he stooped down and wrote on the ground.

At this, those who heard began to go away one at a time, the older ones first, until only Jesus was left, with the woman still standing there. Jesus straightened up and asked her, 'Woman, where are they? Has no one condemned you?'

'No one, sir,' she said.

'Then neither do I condemn you,' Jesus declared. 'Go now and leave your life of sin.'" ~John 8:7-11 (emphasis mine)

Who are we to condemn and ostracize a person whom God Himself has set free and created new? (2 Corinthians 5:17). When we confess our sins and repent of them, the Lord forgives us and casts them as far as the east is from the west (that's pretty darn far!) and remembers them no more (Psalm 103:12, 43:25). Isaiah 38:17 tells us God has put our sins "behind His back"!

If our Father, while in Heaven as the reigning King and also on earth as the sacrificial Lamb of God, extends such mercy and acceptance in spite of our ugly pasts, shouldn't we also show the same love to others, no matter how offensive or off-putting their sins might have been?

Until Christ returns to reign and rule as King on this earth, we are His representatives, His hands, His feet. Let's make every effort to love as He loved during His ministry two-thousand years ago. Let us accept and encourage those He gave His life to forgive and save.

Merciful Father, all the libraries in the world couldn't contain the number of books that could be written on Your magnificent love for us, a love that not only forgives our failures and redeems us from death, but a love that also keeps no record of our countless wrongs. Help us never to forget that we each have strayed and fallen short; we all need grace, love, and forgiveness (Romans 3:23). We ask You to give us hearts that are compassionate and caring, as well as eyes that see beyond a person's past, into their present desire and need for You, not our judgment. We ask this in the Name of Your victorious Son, the conquering King, Jesus, Amen.

WORKOUT 1 — WEEK 16

WARMUP

3 rounds:

- [ ] 10 reverse lunges (5 each leg)
- [ ] 10 high skips (5 each leg)
- [ ] 12 high-kicks (6 each leg)
- [ ] 10 wall squats
- [ ] 15 mock kettlebell swings

WORKOUT BENCHMARK WORKOUT

"Perfect Fit Benchmark 2" (Record results in your "Workout Log") and compare your results with Week 2, Workout 2!

Complete the following in the order given, with proper form:

- [ ] Timed 1 mile run
- [ ] *Rest* 1 minute
- [ ] 2 minutes: as many sit-ups as possible
- [ ] *Rest* 1 minute
- [ ] 2 minutes: as many air squats as possible
- [ ] *Rest* 1 minute
- [ ] 2 minutes: as many push-ups as possible

WORKOUT 2 — WEEK 16

WARMUP

3 rounds:

- [ ] 20 reverse lunges (10 each leg)
- [ ] 5 walk-outs
- [ ] 10 air squats
- [ ] 10 push-ups

WORKOUT

10 minute AMRAP:

- [ ] 5 dumbbell hang-cleans each arm
- [ ] 20 jump rope

AFTERBURN

- [ ] 3 sets of 20 dumbbell bicep curls

WEEK 17

"Blessed be the God and Father of our Lord Jesus Christ, who according to His great mercy has caused us to be born again to a living hope through the resurrection of Jesus Christ from the dead..." ~1 Peter 1:3, NASB

"You earn your body."

"You have to work for the results you want."

"You get out of it when you put into it."

Those and countless other phrases bluntly, yet accurately, describe the ongoing journey to improved health and fitness. As Cher so eloquently stated, "Fitness—If it came in a bottle, everybody would have a great body."

No one, save for comic book superheroes and the genetic, envy-inducing anomalies among us, was born with impeccable health and a flawless body to match. It takes hard work and discipline in the gym and kitchen to both attain and sustain a life permeated with wellness.

Wellness. Merriam-Webster's Dictionary defines it as "the quality or state of being in good health especially as an actively sought goal."

Americans spend $40 **BILLION** a year on weight-loss programs and products.[20] The health club industry is a $20 billion a year business.[21] In 2011, this country spent $10.4 billion on cosmetic surgery, which is more than the gross domestic product of nations such as Chad and Liechtenstein.[22] Wellness (and attractiveness!) certainly is "actively sought!"

Millions of people spend hard-earned money on weight-loss products, diet books, gym memberships, even elective surgeries to eliminate fat or implant muscles and...er, other things. We spend time pushing through tough workouts that elevate our heart rates and break down our muscles so they'll grow back stronger and more powerful. We spend time being sore after killer leg workouts, involuntarily imitating penguins and cowboys with our funny waddles and slow strides. We spend time in uncomfortable stretches, atop fascia-loosening foam rollers and the tables of unforgiving massage therapists to help alleviate that soreness. And when things start to feel easy in a workout, we immediately amp up the intensity to evade the dreaded plateaus that halt our progress. Be it for the sake of vanity or eternity, we're all sweating and spending to *earn* the bodies we want.

As I've been reflecting on Christ's death and resurrection throughout this Easter week, I've been struck not only by the unfathomable depths of the love displayed in his sacrifice, but the immeasurable magnitude of his grace imparted through it:

20 http://www.businessweek.com/debateroom/archives/2008/01/the_diet_indust.html

21 http://www.bizologie.com/the-business-of-staying-fit/

22 http://www.huffingtonpost.com/2012/04/18/plastic-surgery-spending-up-2011_n_1435512.html

"...for all have sinned and fall short of the glory of God, and all are justified freely by his grace through the redemption that came by Christ Jesus." ~Romans 3:23-24, NIV (emphasis mine)

The invitation to have our sins forgiven, our hearts made new, and our hollow, filthy bodies cleansed and filled with God's Holy Spirit is freely sent (Ephesians 2:8, 1 Corinthians 6:19). There is nothing we need do to purchase or provide recompense for such treasures. The fact is, there is nothing we *could* do as thousands of years of diligent law-keeping and devoted sacrifice-making by the Jewish people proved (Gal. 3:21-22, NIV).

The Lord Almighty paid the ultimate price to save you and me when he sent his only Son, the Lamb of God, to perish on a long-prophesied Passover's night over 2,000 years ago.

For those of us who have accepted Jesus Christ as our Lord and Savior, we are promised a glorified body, like Jesus' when he returned to earth for forty days after his resurrection.

"It is sown a natural body; it is raised a spiritual body. If there is a natural body, there is also a spiritual body." ~1 Corinthians 15:44, ESV

With this body, Jesus moved like lightning, able to transport himself from Jerusalem to the two downcast travelers on the Road to Emmaus. And then as quickly as he appeared to them, he vanished from their sight (Luke 24:13-35). Jesus could also pass through material things, which he demonstrated by appearing in the midst of the disciples without opening the door. He also enjoyed food with his resurrected body, cooking and eating a breakfast of bread and fish on the beach with his disciples.

Today we abide in bodies that wrestle with weaknesses and infirmities that God never intended for us. As part of the curse, we toil to tend to them, to keep them healthy and strong, and, morbid as it sounds, to stave off the inevitability of death as best we can.

But one day...

One day we will be clothed immortal, arrayed in robes of radiant white, and the laws of gravity, the limits of time and space, the lust of our flesh, the lies of the enemy will be no more (Revelation 3:4-5, 18). All that cursed creation as a result of the Original Sin will be forgotten as the Holy One wipes every tear from our eyes (Revelation 21:4). Heartache, depression, pain both physical and emotional, even vanity, will dissolve into the glorious light of his love.

I thank God for providing the Way back into his presence after paradise was lost.[23] I thank him for his Son who stepped down from golden streets and angelic praise onto a spinning sphere of sin-cursed soil to save us from our sins. I thank him that one day we will know what true *wellness* really is. I thank him that we will be "just men made perfect," having done nothing but accepting the gift of Yeshua—*Salvation*—to earn such wondrous perfection (Hebrews 12:23).

Loving Abba, Lord you are so good. You are Love and you are Light. You are the Giver of all good gifts. Two-thousand years ago you gave to humanity the greatest gift of all, your only begotten Son, Jesus Christ. Through him we have salvation from our sins, freedom from condemnation, and cures for our broken hearts, troubled minds, and weakened bodies. Through him we arise each day victorious and full of hope because your Word is true and unchanging. Lord, we thank you that our bodies will one day be redeemed. We pray that we will take care of them as best we know how until the day comes that you call us home to Heaven. Help us to honor you today with how we nourish ourselves and exercise, and also by how we conduct ourselves by the actions we take and words we speak. In Jesus' name we pray, Amen.

23 "Paradise Lost" is an epic poem written by John Milton in the 17th century. The poem concerns the biblical Fall of Man as recorded in the Book of Genesis.

WORKOUT 1 — WEEK 17

WARMUP

2 rounds:

- [ ] 200-meter run
- [ ] 8 walk-outs
- [ ] 10 burpees
- [ ] 20 mock kettlebell swings
- [ ] 60 jump rope

WORKOUT

Complete the following as fast as you can with proper form:

4 rounds:

- [ ] 15 box jumps (sub 25 jump squats if you don't have a plyo box)
- [ ] 20 kettlebell swings
- [ ] 200-meter run (0.12 miles)

WORKOUT 2 — WEEK 17

WARMUP

- ☐ 30 lunges (15 each leg)
- ☐ 20 butt-kicks (10 each side)
- ☐ 20 high-knees (10 each side)
- ☐ 20 mountain-climbers (right/left is 1 rep)
- ☐ 20 reverse lunges (10 each leg)
- ☐ 10 broad jumps

WORKOUT

Complete the following as fast as you can with proper form:

- ☐ 100 lunges (50 each leg)
- ☐ 15 burpees
- ☐ 50 sumo deadlift high-pull with kettlebell
- ☐ 15 burpees

AFTERBURN

- ☐ Tabata dips

WEEK 18

*"Consider it a sheer **gift**, friends, when tests and challenges come at you from all sides. You know that **under pressure**, your faith-life is forced into the open and shows its true colors. So don't try to get out of anything prematurely. Let it do its work so you become mature and well-developed, not deficient in any way."* ~James 1:2-4, MSG (emphasis mine)

2 Corinthians 4:7 refers to our bodies as "jars of clay," painting a picture of our perishing state, our frail and feeble condition as a result of sin's stronghold in the earth.

We are all alabaster jars. From jasmine, rose, pine and citrus to cinnamon, sage, and sandalwood, we each contain a unique, God-made, Heaven-bottled fragrance unlike any other wafting through the winds of creation. But like Mary's jar, broken and poured out onto the dusty feet of Jesus, no one will smell the perfume we contain until we've been shattered to release it (Matthew 26:6-13).

Just as new oil is formed using crushed olives, and new wine made by crushing grapes and breaking their skins, the ambrosial blessings within us emerge after we too have endured *tribulation*...

While on the subject of "tribulation," an interesting piece of trivia: The word comes from the Latin word *tribulum,* which is an ancient threshing instrument used in farming. The farmer would stand on it while being pulled by the animal, applying pressure to remove the wheat from the chaff.

Our modern definition of the word "tribulation," according to dictionary.com: "grievous trouble; severe trial or suffering."

I admit, words like "crushing," tribulation," and "suffering" aren't exactly rhetorical rays of sunshine, but I'm encouraged when I read what James, the brother of Jesus, had to say about it:

Whatever the *tribulum* is in your life that's brought you to your knees, whatever the size of the spirit-crushing weight that once rendered you emotionally immobile as you stared up helplessly at a starless sky, let it "do its work" with the Lord's intervention; He wants to anoint it with the supernatural scent of His perfect plan and purpose.

Father, we thank you for Your perfect plan and for the immutable fact that You are able to work all things together for good, as Romans 8:28 assures us. We are so thankful that no trial in our lives, no matter its magnitude, is a surprise to you. You are the Good Shepherd tending to His flock with steadfast provision and unblinking protection. We ask You to give us the wisdom and strength to use the snares, famines, and wolves You've allowed into our pastures and the lessons they've taught us to inspire and encourage others around us with testimonies of Your faithfulness. Help us to trust You completely and remember that in our weaknesses, You are mighty. In the All-Sufficient Name of Jesus we pray, Amen (2 Corinthians 12:9).

WORKOUT 1 — WEEK 18

WARMUP

- [ ] 200-meter jog (0.12 miles)
- [ ] 30 lunges with twist over lunging leg (15 each leg)
- [ ] 20 high-kicks (10 each leg)
- [ ] 20 air squats
- [ ] 10 walk-out/walk-ins
- [ ] 30 jumping jacks
- [ ] 15 jump squats
- [ ] 200-meter run (0.12 miles)

WORKOUT BENCHMARK WORKOUT

"Perfect Fit Benchmark 3" (Record results in your "Workout Log") and compare with the results of Workout 1, Week 4!

Complete the following as fast as you can with proper form:

- [ ] 100 alternating lunges
- [ ] 100 sit-ups
- [ ] 50 push-ups
- [ ] 50 squats

WORKOUT 2 — WEEK 18

WARMUP

- [ ] 400-meter jog
- [ ] 10 walk-outs
- [ ] 30 butt-kicks (15 each leg)
- [ ] 30 forward arm circles
- [ ] 30 reverse arm circles
- [ ] 20 arm swings (backward/forward is 1 rep)
- [ ] 20 jumping jacks

WORKOUT

11 minute AMRAP:

- [ ] 6 double-unders (sub 18 single jump ropes if unable to do double-unders)
- [ ] 7 pull-ups (sub bent-over dumbbell rows if you don't have a pull-up bar)
- [ ] 8 suit-case deadlifts

AFTERBURN

- [ ] 25 burpees for time

WEEK 19

By   Colleen Long

Age   31

Occupation Registered Sales Assistant and Owner of Sew.
            Thread. Ink.

"For my thoughts are not your thoughts, neither are your ways my ways," declares the Lord. As the heavens are higher than the earth, so are my ways higher than your ways and my thoughts than your thoughts" ~Isaiah 55:8-10, NIV

Until recently, I did not have a true appreciation for God's design, nor wisdom regarding His work of preparation and timing in our lives.

A few months ago, I was in a car accident. I was on my way home from Bible study, and as I was waiting to pull into my driveway, someone rear-ended me going 55 miles per hour. My car was totaled and I suffered head, neck, and back injuries. I was left with a severe concussion that affected my day-to-day activities for several weeks. I thank God He spared my life because the accident could have been much worse. That night and the weeks that followed opened my eyes to God's sovereign handiwork of preparation and timing in my life.

Six months prior to my wreck, I did workouts at my CrossFit gym. Even during my college days as a soccer player, I never experienced anything close to what I have experienced with my workout family; I loved the hard work and the results I was feeling and seeing even more. Just before starting at the CrossFit gym, I went gluten-free and was very intentional with the types of foods I ate and prepared for my husband and myself. Two years before going gluten-free, I had begun chiropractic care. All of those decisions to honor God through stewardship for my body led me to be in the best shape I have ever been in my life. I was incredibly discouraged when my accident happened because I had worked so hard and made so much progress physically. I saw the accident as a major setback…but God graciously showed me otherwise.

The day after my accident, I went to my chiropractor for an examination. They took X-rays of my neck, and it was very evident that it was worse than when I had my first visit.

My initial thought was: *Two years worth of chiropractic care down the drain.*

Then the Holy Spirit opened my eyes and I realized something: the adjustments didn't go to waste! God knew that I was going to be in this accident long ago, and over time He was strengthening and preparing my body to withstand the impact. I could have been seriously injured or even broken my neck from the accident if I had not been actively pursuing a healthy lifestyle. God's timing and design to use positive health changes in my life—although they were just daily choices and activities—were tools that God used to save my life. Praise God for His omniscience!

During those weeks of recovery, I gained a new perspective on God's timing. The timing of the accident reminded me of the fragility of life. The timing of my training and other health choices I'd made reminded me of how the Lord blesses those who seek to honor Him and how He guides our steps. The timing of our met needs after the accident reminded me of how vital the Body of Christ is, and that we genuinely need one another. The timing of God's healing and the road to recovery, although I did not know how long it would take, reminded me that if the Lord could spare my life from the accident, then He could heal me too.

Even though we do not always understand what God is doing or why, we do know that He is good, that He is eternally wise, and that He loves us beyond measure. God always directs our steps, whether or not we recognize or acknowledge His handiwork. His timing is always perfect, and if He has the power to eternally save you, He can surely sustain you through all things in life.

"Yet God has made everything beautiful for its own time. He has planted eternity in the human heart, but even so, people cannot see the whole scope of God's work from beginning to end. So I concluded there is nothing better than to be happy and enjoy ourselves as long as we can. And people should eat and drink and enjoy the fruits of their labor, for these are gifts from God. And I know that whatever God does is final. Nothing can be added to it or taken from it. God's purpose is that people should fear him. What is happening now has happened before, and what will happen in the future has happened before, because God makes the same things happen over and over again." ~Ecclesiastes 3:11-15, NLT

Dear Jesus, thank you that you are our Sovereign King and that You are in control of all things at all times. Help us to trust Your timing, to respect Your ways, and to enjoy the gift of life that You have died for us to live. May we rest and celebrate in Your wisdom knowing that You have a plan and purpose for our lives. Grant us the strength live a life of faith as an example to those around us. Keep us in Your will, Father, and may we grow more in love with You day by day. We pray this in Jesus' name, by whose grace we are able to do all things. Amen.

WORKOUT 1 — WEEK 19

WARMUP

2 rounds:

☐ 20 butt-kicks (10 each leg)

☐ 20 high-knees (1o each leg)

☐ 20 mountain-climbers (right/left = 1 rep)

☐ 15 air squats

☐ 15 push-ups

☐ 5 burpees

WORKOUT

Complete the following as fast as you can, maintaining proper form:

1-2-3-4-5-6-7-8-9-10 with 100-meter run (0.06 miles) between sets:

☐ Goblet squats with kettlebell

AFTERBURN

☐ Tabata split-squats (alternating right and left legs with each set)

WORKOUT 2 — WEEK 19

WARMUP

- [ ] 20 lunges each leg
- [ ] 10 high skips (5 each leg)
- [ ] 20 butt-kicks (10 each leg)
- [ ] 20 high-knees (10 each leg)
- [ ] 200-meter (0.12 mile run)
- [ ] 10 air squats
- [ ] 20 arm circles forward
- [ ] 20 arm circles backwards
- [ ] 10 push-ups

WORKOUT BENCHMARK WORKOUT

"Perfect Fit Benchmark 4" (Record results in your "Workout Log") and compare with results of Workout 1, Week 5!

Complete the following three rounds as fast as you can with proper form:

- [ ] 800-meter run (0.5 miles)
- [ ] 15 dumbbell thrusters

WEEK 20

"Let no corrupting talk come out of your mouths, but only such as is good for building up, as fits the occasion, that it may give grace to those who hear" ~Ephesians 4:29, ESV

"Again, being a part of this community is the best reason to join CrossFit 925!"

That was the recent Facebook status of one of the athletes we coach at CrossFit 925 posted just hours after our box closed up for the night after hosting the first workout of the 2013 CrossFit Open for our athletes. How awesome is it that "community" can be considered the foremost reason to embark upon a fitness lifestyle?!

Last Friday night, twenty-five competitors divided among five heats went up against workout 13.1, a physically and mentally try-ing seventeen-minute AMRAP that tested each athlete's strength and stamina. For two and half hours, people of all ages and fitness levels took turns "burpeeing" and snatching side by side, giving every ounce of strength and drop of sweat they had to find out how many reps they could achieve as the clock counted down.[24]

And when athletes weren't competing in the workout, they were cheering…*loudly*…

There's a popular and proven stereotype in the CrossFit community which holds that the athletes in last place receive the most cheers. Our box took that slogan one step further during Friday's workout, demonstrating that those who are struggling and battling frustration most cause the walls to shake and roof to be raised with the high-spirited shouts of encouragement they elicit.

I'll take myself as an example. I completed my burpees and the lighter set of snatches (forty-five pounds) in ten minutes, thirty seconds. I had over six minutes to see how many reps of seventy-five-pound snatches I could do. Considering the heaviest I've ever snatched is eighty pounds, I told myself beforehand that I would be elated if I could pull off just one seventy-five-pound snatch that night.

For nearly five minutes, I tried and failed, tried and failed, tried and failed. But the entire time, athletes and supportive onlookers were cheering me on: *"Go, Diana! You can do it! You got this!"* They simply wouldn't stop cheering. They wouldn't lose hope. They kept it up until I finally accomplished one rep. And with ten seconds left on the clock, I did a second rep, surpassing my goal.[25] With all of the clapping and celebration pervading the chalk-filled atmosphere, you'd have thought I'd just won gold at the Olympics. And I felt as though I had.

---

24 The snatch is a complex Olympic lifting movement, the goal of which is to lift a barbell from the ground to locked arms overhead in a smooth and continuous movement.

25 A few hours ago, I did this workout again and did five reps better than the first time. This further proves that the confidence others place in us can lift us up and carry us great distances.

The Bible says life and death are in the power of the tongue (Proverbs 18:21). We all know how devastating words can be. They can rip apart relationships, fracture friendships, and decimate dreams. They can produce doubt, create lies, perpetuate rumors, and shatter confidence in a few easy breaths. But words can also be life-givers and resuscitators.

Words have the power to move an athlete past her frustrations to a personal peak of victory. They have the power to call a dead man from the tomb and to dress dry bones with flesh (John 11:44, Ezekiel 37). And whether spoken to you or by you, they can transform your situation, redeem your day, and rejuvenate your life.

I honestly don't believe that I could have moved that bar over my head had it not been for the confidence-boosting, perseverance-promoting, and exhilaration-inducing encouragement of these wonderful people. Without their voices pushing me to keep going, to keep striving, I would have given up and walked away with minutes still running on the clock. I was marvelously blessed and indeed, built up, by the cheers they provided, for they were a perfect fit for the occasion.

"The words of the reckless pierce like swords, but the tongue of the wise brings healing." ~Proverbs 12:18, NIV

Dear Father of Lights, Creator of all beauty, Author of all truth, we praise you for our brothers and sisters in Christ who build us up when we feel low, who speak encouragement when we feel depressed, who believe in our success when we feel like failures. Help us today to open our hearts to the grace-giving cheers of others and to look for opportunities to cheer up the discouraged and downcast around us. Help us to cast off corruptive words and the festering thoughts that cripple and bind us and to speak only words that produce life, words full of grace and hope and love. It is in Jesus' sweet-sounding, life-giving, soul-saving name we pray, Amen.

WORKOUT 1 — WEEK 20

WARMUP

2 rounds:

- [ ] 20 butt-kicks (10 each leg)
- [ ] 20 high-knees (1o each leg)
- [ ] 20 mountain-climbers (right/left = 1 rep)
- [ ] 15 air squats
- [ ] 15 push-ups
- [ ] 5 burpees

WORKOUT

Complete the following as fast as you can, with proper form, in the order given:

- [ ] 75 jumping jacks
- [ ] 75 air squats
- [ ] 75 sit-ups
- [ ] 50 dumbbell squats
- [ ] 50 weighted sit-ups
- [ ] 50 jumping jacks

WORKOUT 2 — WEEK 20

WARMUP

- ☐ 400-meter jog
- ☐ 10 walk-outs
- ☐ 20 arm circles forward
- ☐ 20 arm circles reverse
- ☐ 20 mountain-climbers (right/left is 1 rep)
- ☐ 20 air squats
- ☐ 10 burpees

WORKOUT

15 minute AMRAP:

- ☐ 5 chin-ups (sub bent-over, underhanded dumbbell rows if you don't have a pull-up bar)
- ☐ 10 decline push-ups (if you don't have a box, you can place feet on the edge of sturdy bench, chair, even a sofa!)
- ☐ 200-meter run

WEEK 21

"Make a careful exploration of who you are and the work you have been given, and then sink yourself into that. Don't be impressed with yourself. Don't compare yourself with others. Each of you must take responsibility for doing the creative best you can with your own life"
~Galatians 6:4-5, MSG

As a CrossFit coach, each day I am blessed with the opportunity to help men and women get one step closer to their goals. Whether it's improving stamina, gaining strength, losing weight, or attaining greater energy levels, I am continuously inspired by the progress each athlete makes. There are days, however, when I lose sight of my personal goals and successes and instead focus on and envy what others have, be it their ability to perform a heavier clean and jerk or their faster "Angie" time.[26]

---

26 "Angie" is a benchmark workout in CrossFit. We typically do this WOD (workout of the day) once every three or four months to monitor our progress. This particular timed WOD consists of doing 100 pull-ups, 100 push-ups, 100 sit-ups, and 100 squats as fast as you can.

Proverbs 14:30 says that a peaceful heart gives life to the body, but envy rots the bones. When we allow our admiration of others' gifts, blessings, beauty and strength to morph into jealousy, we stray from our God-carved path in pursuit of someone else's. By complaining and comparing ourselves to those around us, we show a lack of trust in the One who's promised to prosper us, not to harm us, the One who has entrusted to us gifts as unique as our fingerprints, gifts meant to thrive and flourish for a tailor-made purpose (Jeremiah 29:11, 1 Peter 4:10).

Rather than looking at your friend and wishing you had her legs, her job, her artistic talent, her sense of humor, etc., praise God for the blessings He's given you. Start with His Son, Your Savior, and work your way down the list to whatever talent you have that you know is God-given. Then focus on doing your best and giving your all in the job, workout, or class you're in right now! The inclination to compare yourself with anyone else will vanish as you feel the satisfaction and security of knowing that God is pleased with you.

"For am I now seeking the approval of man, or of God? Or am I trying to please man? If I were still trying to please man, I would not be a servant of Christ." ~Galatians 1:10, ESV

Dear Lord, we praise Your eternal Name. We thank You for loving us with an unfailing, unconditional love, a love that blesses us daily with our every need and reaches down to us continually with comforting rays of light and grace, peace and compassion. We ask forgiveness for failing to praise You when we ought. Instead of thinking on and thanking You for the abundant blessings You've rained down on us, we so often turn to others and compare ourselves with envy. Help us to be confident in who we are as children of the Living God and joyful for what we have as co-heirs with Your Son, Jesus. Help us to derive our satisfaction and joy from our identity in Christ. Let it be our pleasure and passion to bring glory to His name with our specially crafted gifts and talents. Let Your will be done in us, Lord. In the Name of Jesus, the One we strive to serve with the time we've been given, Amen.

WORKOUT 1 — WEEK 21

WARMUP

3 rounds:

- [ ] 10 high-skips (5 each side)
- [ ] 20 butt-kicks (20 each side)
- [ ] 20 high-knees (20 each side)
- [ ] 100 meter run (0.06 miles)
- [ ] 20 scorpions (10 each side)
- [ ] 10 jump squats

WORKOUT

Complete the following as fast as you can, maintaining proper form:

- [ ] 1,000-meter run (0.6 miles)
- [ ] 100 air squats
- [ ] 90 lunges (45 each leg)
- [ ] 80 sit-ups
- [ ] 60 double-unders (or 180 singles if unable to do double-unders)

WORKOUT 2 — WEEK 21

WARMUP

3 rounds:

- [ ] 10 reverse lunges (5 each leg)
- [ ] 10 high skips (5 each leg)
- [ ] 20 high-kicks (10 each leg)
- [ ] 10 wall squats
- [ ] 15 mock kettlebell swings

WORKOUT

5 minute AMREP:

- [ ] Burpees
- [ ] *Rest* 2 minutes.
- [ ] 4 minute AMREP
- [ ] Kettlebell swings

WEEK 22

By   Lynda Schmidt
Age   45
Occupation Nurse Practitioner for a Bariatric Surgeon

"I have given you authority to trample on snakes and scorpions and to overcome all the power of the enemy; nothing will harm you" ~Luke 10:19, NIV

I began working out at my CrossFit gym about 2 months after I began my new job working for a Bariatric surgeon. Needless to say, the two go hand in hand; I teach my patients about diet and exercise and tout the advantages of high-intensity training on a daily basis.

About a year after I began training at my gym, I entered the competition arena. Now that I have about five competitions and one trip to the CrossFit Games Regionals competition under my belt, I feel like I am doing pretty well. I never thought that I would be in the best shape of my life at age forty-five!

By competing individually as part of a team, I've taken myself out of my comfort zone and stepped into the closest thing to a spotlight I've personally ever experienced. I've struggled with this because I am not used to people telling me that I inspire them or that they wish they could do the things I do. I think to myself: *"I'm just working out and enjoying getting stronger."*

I began to ask how I could give glory back to the One who was giving it to me. How could I turn the spotlight, if you will, back to Jesus? Why, a tattoo of course! So I thought long and hard. I came up with several ideas, but none of them were quite right.

The day I received my "tattoo epiphany" was while I was talking to my priest. I explained that I did not want to be prideful of my body or the gifts I had been given that allow me to participate in the sport of CrossFit.

While we were talking I had a vision of the Archangel Michael. That was it! That's the tattoo I wanted! Who better than the Archangel Michael? After all, he must have been pretty "Beast" to throw Satan out of Heaven! He is absolutely the Warrior for Christ.

I became so convicted that I called my tattoo artist that evening and made an appointment. I remember telling him, "I want the Archangel Michael, but you have to make him ripped and strong. He has to be tough. I want people to know that I am a warrior for Christ."

The very next day I went back to the box after taking a week-long break before starting to train hard for the Games. I warmed up as usual and went to work. The "Strength" routine for the day was three sets, three reps each of front squats. I felt pretty confident. The heaviest front squat I could perform for one repetition was 155 pounds, so I began with ninety-five and did a few warm-up sets. I loaded the bar for my first of three heavy reps, trying to work my way up to 160 pounds. Suffice it to say, I never got there…

I started my first set of three and *WHAM!* As I was standing up after the first squat, my hamstring "popped." I dropped the weight and went to the ground. I was devastated. What now? The Games were three months away. I couldn't even do a basic air squat.

It was very strange. I had told my coach that morning about the epiphany that I'd had regarding my tattoo and how I wanted to be a warrior for Christ. My coach is a very godly man, and he had been training me for months to get to this place. He came to me after the workout was over, after I'd rolled and stretched and iced to alleviate the pain. He said:

"You know this is the devil trying to take your conviction away, don't you? Why do you think he chose today to test you?"

I contemplated what my coach had said. He was absolutely right. *If I truly want to be a warrior for Christ I have to overcome this,* I thought. We prayed for healing soon after.

I began doing some light exercising and stretching to get back at it. I did a lot more upper body and gymnastic movements to keep me going. Finally the day I was waiting for came, the day I'd get my tattoo! But then came the disappointing e-mail. My tattoo artist had a death in the family and said we would have to delay my appointment for another two weeks. I was upset, but of course understood.

I'm not sure exactly when I had the dream, but it is so vivid to me. I dreamt that I was being pursued by a gigantic snake. It was chasing me down the street, and I was terrified, as you can imagine. But all of a sudden, I thought, *Why am I running?*

So I turned around and I grabbed the snake by the throat—if snake's have throats—and I remember thinking, *Just leave me alone and I will let you go.* Then the snake bit me on my hand. I didn't let go. Instead, I ripped its head off with my bare hands!

My "dream self" then thought, *Okay, great, now I have to get to an emergency room and get treated for this venomous bite.*

Of course we all know how dreams are. If you're trying to get somewhere, you NEVER get there. Through the course of the dream, I realized my hand was healing and getting better. I didn't need to go to the emergency room after all. That snake wasn't so bad. I conquered it!

I relayed this dream to my coach. He said immediately, "That was you conquering Satan, you can beat this injury and stay on track."

So finally, the day came for my appointment. I'd been waiting for what seemed like an eternity and was so excited to see what my tattoo artist had drawn up for me. I arrived to the shop and he said, "Lynda, I've got something in mind, but it's not exactly the Archangel Michael. I have done that tattoo so many times. I want yours to be unique."

He pulled the piece of paper he had sketched my design on out of the folder. It was a magnificent, fierce-looking lion with huge wings, and under his front paw was a serpent. Every muscle was defined, and the look on the lion's face was one of pure rage.

I looked at it, and remarked that that wasn't really what I'd had in mind. I was imagining something a bit more feminine and not nearly as big and bold. I felt like he really hadn't heard what I had told him. Then he said, "I have been praying about this piece for about a month now, and the Scripture that came to me is: Luke 10:19 which says, 'Behold, I give unto you power to tread on serpents and scorpions, and over all the power of the enemy: and nothing shall by any means hurt you.'"

I literally got goose bumps. A chill traveled down my spine! I then proceeded to tell him about the dream from the week before. He couldn't believe it.

Needless to say, I now have a very large, very fierce lion tattoo on my side.

I believe that the Lord speaks to us all in different ways. Sometimes they are not as conventional as we would like them to be, but I couldn't ignore this. My hope is that people will see this tattoo and ask me what it represents.

My gym is a wonderful community. We share defeat, victory, pain, and laughter. But there are a great number of us that feel we grow spiritually as well as physically when we train and compete. Giving our all and sharing that experience with others somehow brings us closer to Christ and to those around us in ways that are mysterious and awe-inspiring. I see those of us with this conviction as warriors for Christ. Through our faith and zeal for the Lord, we show others Who it we live for and why we strive to honor our bodies and clothe it with strength (Proverbs 31:25).

Great God in Heaven, Father of the Lion of the Tribe of Judah, we thank you that we have victory through Jesus to overcome any scorpion in our path and every serpent that pursues us. You have crushed the head of the Old Serpent Satan through Jesus' atoning work on the cross and will one day throw him into the lake of burning sulfur (Revelation 20:10). While we wrestle with evil powers and principalities in this life, we are more than conquerors through Christ and thank you for your promises to protect us, guide us, and grant us victory if we would simply place our trust in you (Romans 8:37). Help us to always give glory to you for our gifts, our achievements, and our victories, for we know we cannot do one good thing of any eternal significance apart from you. We pray these things in your Son's almighty, death-defeating name, Amen.

WORKOUT 1 — WEEK 22

WARMUP

- ☐ 20 lunges each leg
- ☐ 10 high skips (5 each leg)
- ☐ 20 butt-kicks (10 each leg)
- ☐ 20 high-knees (10 each leg)
- ☐ 200-meter (0.12 mile run)
- ☐ 10 wall squats
- ☐ 20 arm circles forward
- ☐ 20 arm circles backwards
- ☐ 10 push-ups

WORKOUT

20 minute AMRAP:

- ☐ 20 suitcase deadlifts
- ☐ 10 dumbbell push-press
- ☐ 20 sit-ups
- ☐ 100-meter run

WORKOUT 2 — WEEK 22

WARMUP

- [ ] 200-meter jog
- [ ] 10 walk-out/walk-ins
- [ ] 20 scorpions (10 each side)
- [ ] 20 wall squats
- [ ] 20 sit-ups to toe-reaches
- [ ] 40 jumping jacks

WORKOUT

Complete the following as fast as you can with proper form:[27]

- [ ] 12-9-6-3 pull-ups (Substitute bent-over dumbbell rows if you don't have a pull-up bar with bands to assist you, or you don't have access to a gym with an assisted pull-up machine.)
- [ ] 3-6-9-12 box jumps (sub broad jumps if you don't have a box)

AFTERBURN

- [ ] 400-meter run for time.

---

27 Perform 12 pull-ups, then 3 jumps. Then do 9 pull-ups, followed by 6 jumps. In other words, alternate between the two exercises.

WEEK 23

"For this light momentary affliction is preparing for us an eternal weight of glory beyond all comparison" ~2 Corinthians 4:17, ESV

This past Sunday at church, pastor and author Max Lucado touched on the joy-filling, hope-stirring subject of heaven. He dispelled the farcical notion that in Paradise, we'll spend eternity on an ethereal cloud bank nestled somewhere between Neptune and Never Never Land, strumming harps whilst naked, winged infants float nearby like Renaissance-era Cupids. Mr. Lucado quoted God's Word to assure us that in fact, Heaven will be much more homey and familiar than we might expect. It will be a glorified *earth…*

"The wolf will live with the lamb,
the leopard will lie down with the goat,
the calf and the lion and the yearling together;
and a little child will lead them.
The cow will feed with the bear,
their young will lie down together,
and the lion will eat straw like the ox.
The infant will play near the cobra's den,
and the young child will put its hand into the viper's nest.
They will neither harm nor destroy
on all my holy mountain,
for the earth will be filled with the knowledge of the Lord
as the waters cover the sea." -Isaiah 11:6-19 (NIV)

Far from a mystical, moonlight haze populated with Kumba-ya-humming transparent bodies and fat, flying babies, heaven will look the way God intended it to, like the pristine and perfect Garden of Eden before Adam and Eve succumbed to temptation.

Mr. Lucado calls our vapor of a life on this earth a "warm-up" for our eternal life on the glorified earth. As a CrossFit coach, I naturally think of things like butt-kicks and high-knees when I hear the word "warm-up." Warm-ups aren't exactly the most popular part of the workout for most people. Stiff muscles don't like the feel of a full range of motion. Sleepy eyes at 5:15 in the morning or 6:30 at night don't like the sight of "100 jump rope" and "400-meter run" written on our "Dynamic Warm-up" board. Fortunately, all of our athletes know how critical the warm-up is to their main workout, so complaints are kept to a minimum! If you aren't aware, here are a few warm-up benefits that I hope encourage you to do the ones contained in this book:

- Elevation of body temperature
- Increase blow flow in the muscles
- Improves efficient cooling
- Improves range of motion
- Reduces incidence and likelihood of musculoskeletal injuries
- Supplies adequate blood flow to heart
- Provides rehearsal of movements present in the workout
- Mental preparation

As you can see, the warm-up prepares us for an effective and rewarding workout. When the workout (the fun part!) begins, our blood is flowing hot, our hearts are pumping strong, and our minds are thinking fast; each part of us giving one-hundred percent to the exercises at hand.

Life on this earth really is like a warm-up. Some days we wake up feeling too tired, too stiff, too anxious to get moving. Sometimes the list of exercises written on the "Dynamic Warm-Up" board of our lives seems endless. So often are the benefits promised to arise from our faithfulness forgotten when we focus only on the "light and momentary afflictions" that have tainted the groaning remnants of Eden (2 Corinthians 4:17, Romans 8:22).

So what's the solution? How do we silence the grumbling and complaining and banish bad attitudes? We must turn to Christ, the One who endured the greatest turmoil, disappointment, and pain of any human in history because He focused His heart heavenward.

"...fixing our eyes on Jesus, the pioneer and perfecter of faith. For the joy set before him he endured the cross, scorning its shame, and sat down at the right hand of the throne of God."
~Hebrews 12:2, NIV

This warm-up isn't easy, but as Paul wrote, it is "nothing compared to the glory" that is to come when our eyes are at last thrilled with the appearance of our Savior's face (Romans 8:17-18).

Lord in Heaven, we thank you for this day and praise you for the hope we have, that at the end of our days, we will look into Jesus' eyes and walk with Him as you walked with Adam and Eve in Eden. Help us keep our hearts and minds fixed on Heaven. Help us to warm up strong and run our race hard, giving this life everything we've got, knowing that we do it all for an eternal Kingdom and its most glorious, loving, and praiseworthy King. Help us not to let bad attitudes and complaints invade and corrupt our days. When we're tempted to let anxiety overtake us, bring quickly to our minds verses like today's which remind us that our most terrible troubles today are nothing in comparison with the wondrous glory and joys to come. In Jesus' holy name, Amen.

WORKOUT 1 — WEEK 23

WARMUP

3 rounds:

- [ ] 200-meter jog (0.12 miles)
- [ ] 30 air squats
- [ ] 5 walk-outs
- [ ] 10 high skips (5 each leg)
- [ ] 20 butt-kicks (10 each leg)
- [ ] 20 high-knees (10 each leg)
- [ ] 5 burpees

WORKOUT

Complete the following as fast as you can, maintaining proper form:

2 rounds:

- [ ] 24 dumbbell thrusters
- [ ] 20 oblique twists with dumbbell (10 each side)
- [ ] 400-meter run

WORKOUT 2 — WEEK 23

WARMUP

2 rounds:

- ☐ 20 reverse lunges (10 each leg)
- ☐ 15 air squats
- ☐ 20 lunges with oblique twist (10 each leg)
- ☐ 10 high skips (5 each side)
- ☐ 10 scorpions (5 each side)

WORKOUT

16 minute AMRAP:

- ☐ 10 dumbbell hang-clean and jerk (5 each arm)
- ☐ 12 bent-over dumbbell row
- ☐ 14 push-ups

WEEK 24

"What are mere mortals that you should think about them, human beings that you should care for them?" ~Psalm 8:4, NLT

I wrote in my book *Fit for Faith* that I received a true revelation the night I read 1 Peter 5:7 with wet, tear-stung eyes and a desperate heart longing for a breakthrough regarding my eating disorder. The verse tells us to cast all of our cares and anxieties upon God because he cares for us. For the first time in my life, I decided to trust God and consequently asked Him to carry *all* of my burdens; I realized not only is there nothing too big for Him to handle, there's nothing *too small* for Him to care about.

Jesus told us that our Father knows when a sparrow falls (Matthew 10:29). He feeds the birds (Matthew 6:26). It should go without saying that He is infinitely more interested in feeding His children and helping us fly again than He is looking after our feathered friends. How blessed we are to serve a God who not only knows how many hairs cover our heads, but also loves us enough to help us with our every struggle, be it in a relationship, a college course, a family illness, or an eating disorder (Luke 12:7).

It's exceedingly difficult for us to wrap our minds around the concept of eternity, let alone the fact that God had us—you and me—in mind since the beginning…whenever that was (Jeremiah 1:5, Ephesians 1:4)! Our parents only had nine months to imagine us before we were born and to prepare for our arrival into this world. God had <u>millennia</u> on top of millennia to plan a life for you, a life filled with His peace, power, and presence if we would place our trust in His Son, Jesus (John 10:10).

Remember throughout your day today that not only does God see you, He cares deeply for you! He spent just as much time designing you as He did the wings of the beautiful Monarch butterfly, the feathers of the majestic peacock, and the countless fish of all colors, shapes, and sizes traversing the seas. He loves you as an artist loves His masterpiece and as a good daddy loves His child. Turn to Him with your worries. Let Him give you wisdom that the world cannot provide. You won't be disappointed. You'll never be turned away.

"For the foolishness of God is wiser than man's wisdom, and the weakness of God is stronger than man's strength." ~1 Corinthians 1:25, NIV

Father God, how grateful we are that despite our microscopic size in the grand scheme of the galaxies, You are mindful of us. Despite our many flaws and daily failures, You love and accept us because You sent Your only Son to die for our sins. We ask You today to help us love you as a bride loves her groom and to cry out to You as a child cries out to its daddy. In Jesus' holy Name, Amen.

WORKOUT 1 — WEEK 24

WARMUP

3 rounds:

- [ ] 10 reverse lunges (5 each leg)
- [ ] 10 high skips (5 each leg)
- [ ] 12 high-kicks (6 each leg)
- [ ] 10 wall squats
- [ ] 15 mock kettlebell swings

WORKOUT

Complete the following as fast as you can with proper form:

- [ ] 21-15-9 box jumps (sub broad jumps if you don't have a box)
- [ ] Weighted sit-ups with dumbbell
- [ ] Kettlebell swings

AFTERBURN

- [ ] 3 sets of 200-meter run (0.12 miles). Rest 1 minute between sets.

WORKOUT 2 — WEEK 24

WARMUP

- [ ] 400-meter jog
- [ ] 10 walk-outs
- [ ] 30 butt-kicks (15 each leg)
- [ ] 30 forward arm circles
- [ ] 30 reverse arm circles
- [ ] 20 arm swings (backward/forward is 1 rep)
- [ ] 20 jumping jacks

WORKOUT

Complete the following as fast as you can, maintaining proper form:

- [ ] 10 burpees
- [ ] 15 v-ups
- [ ] 100 jump rope
- [ ] 15 burpees
- [ ] 10 v-ups
- [ ] 100 jump rope
- [ ] 20 burpees
- [ ] 5 v-ups
- [ ] 100 jump rope

WEEK 25

"Then, because so many people were coming and going that they did not even have a chance to eat, he said to them, 'Come with me by yourselves to a quiet place and get some rest'" ~Mark 6:31, NIV

As a trainer, I'm constantly bugging my clients about their nutrition...whether they like it or not! If one of the ladies I coach in the morning says she's feeling nauseous or lightheaded mid-way through the warm-up, I'll ask: "Did you eat enough for breakfast?"

Often the reply is something like this: "I had a hectic morning getting the kids up and ready for school and didn't have time to eat. I had a bite of my child's waffle and a sip of orange juice before we left." Not exactly the breakfast of champions!

Those who seem to be lagging in the evening classes confess to not having eaten since lunch, which could have been up to six hours earlier! Their reasons: *I didn't have a chance to eat,* or, *I got busy and just forgot!*

By now, our athletes at CrossFit 925 realize the importance of making time for snacks and respectable meals, even preparing them before work to carry with them throughout the day so that by the time they hit the gym, the feel strong, focused, and energized.

But trainers and coaches aren't the only ones concerned about proper nutrition. Jesus is, too! After traveling around in pairs, ministering to people and healing them of demons and diseases, the twelve disciples were exhausted...and hungry! Jesus, being both Creator and man, knew better than anyone that these men needed a little *R and R*. *Olive Garden* the restaurant might not have been around yet, but I like to think they made it to a nearby olive grove and had a picnic.

Getting away to a "quiet place" is not just a trendy tip touted by fitness magazines and celebrity doctors; the Great Physician gave this prescription for revitalization over two-thousand years ago. As you go about your day today, remember to carve a few minutes from your calendar to turn off the world around you. Silence your phone and set it aside. Put your computer to sleep for a few minutes and shut your office door. Refuel your body with a healthy snack and feed your spirit with life-sustaining Scripture from God's Word. No matter how busy you are, you'll never regret setting time aside to be alone with the One who loves to be with you more than anyone.

Dear Lord, we thank You for another day, a day filled with people we love, jobs to do that glorify You and show the world Your grace, and strength to live a healthy life on fire for Your Son. We ask You to guide us today and nudge us into a quiet place with You where we can receive rest and refreshment in the incomparable presence of the Prince of Peace. Help us never to let the busyness of life supersede sacred time alone with You. In Jesus' Name we pray, Amen.

WORKOUT 1 — WEEK 25

WARMUP

2 rounds:

- ☐ 20 butt-kicks (10 each leg)
- ☐ 20 high-knees (1o each leg)
- ☐ 20 mountain-climbers (right/left = 1 rep)
- ☐ 15 wall squats
- ☐ 15 push-ups
- ☐ 5 burpees

WORKOUT

5 minute AMREP :

- ☐ 200-meter run
- ☐ Max air squats
- ☐ *Rest* 1 minute.

3 minute AMREP:

- ☐ 200-meter run
- ☐ Max box jumps (do squat jumps if you don't have a box)

AFTERBURN

- ☐ 50 mountain-climbers for time.

WORKOUT 2 — WEEK 25

WARMUP

- ☐ 400-meter jog
- ☐ 10 walk-outs
- ☐ 20 arm circles forward
- ☐ 20 arm circles reverse
- ☐ 20 high-kicks (10 each leg)
- ☐ 20 mountain-climbers (right/left is 1 rep)
- ☐ 20 air squats
- ☐ 10 burpees

WORKOUT

Complete the following as fast as you can with proper form:

3 rounds:

- ☐ 30 suitcase deadlifts
- ☐ 10 sit-ups
- ☐ 10 dumbbell strict press

AFTERBURN

- ☐ 50 renegade rows (25 each arm)

WEEK 26

By   Susan Dotter
Age   43
Occupation Speech therapist

"Therefore we do not lose heart. Though outwardly we are wasting away, yet inwardly we are being renewed day by day. For our light and momentary troubles are achieving for us an eternal glory that far outweighs them all. So we fix our eyes not on what is seen, but on what is unseen, since what is seen is temporary, but what is unseen is eternal"
~2 Corinthians 4:16-18, NIV

Time passes so quickly. We look up and that cute little toddler in the smocked dress with the turned-down anklet socks is driving off in the car with your three other precious children in it. The reflection in the mirror has those same little lines around her eyes that remind us of our parents' faces. Everyone tells you this will happen but somehow even though we are aware, time seems to zip by, leaving our hair blowing and our breath heaving from the hurried and scurried pace at which we often live.

Some days I move so quickly through the day, I swear my lips feel chapped from the whizzing and zipping that goes on in and out of carpool lines. (Okay, maybe that's because I forgot to take time to drink enough water and replenish my body, but you get my meaning, right?). A clock or handheld device buzzes, dings, or even sings to let us know what's next, what's coming, or at times, what we inadvertently missed!

Don't get me wrong, I am completely and totally reliant on said devices and am in no way advocating that we go without mindfulness of our schedules and tasks of the day. But what I wish to emphasize is that we shouldn't be stressed out and let our minds worry and wonder about the tasks of the day. God has a way of giving us respite from this hurried pace if we only allow him to. He reminds us in his Word that time is fleeting, that our earthly home with all of the soccer practices, traffic jams, and business meetings that go too long and make us miss our flight are temporary. Yet, somehow, even though we know things are temporary, we allow them to dictate our attitude about how we will get through it. Imagine what could happen if we began to view our days through the lens of *temporary*...not in an effort to negate its worth but to really value what God gives us in it.

What if we wait expectantly, excitedly, and readily for the time when we join him? I'm not talking about not participating, nor am I downplaying the importance of carpools and grocery lists. I'm talking about looking at what God is giving us in the moment and imagining how much he loves us in it and through it! That traffic jam you are sitting in? Imagine if you were that fellow on the side of the road with the backpack, longing for a car of his own. What if we decided to use that time to talk with God about our day, finding and reflecting on the blessings he has graciously given us? That

PTA meeting with its varied personalities may be our opportunity to learn from others and allow God to teach us to love others as he does.

What if...just what if...that exercise class we've been meaning to go to is filled with God's perfect friendships for you on your journey to better health? What if as we sweat and huff, and puff, we are mindful of the fact that the pain is temporary? What if we look ahead of us as we jog along on our path and think of the steps we took before that brought us thus far rather than dreading the ones that lie ahead?

It's all temporary. It may be hard, it might not be fun, and you might even hate it at times! But, the reward...oh, the reward that awaits us as we keep our eyes on Him! I encourage you to view whatever your struggle is through a mindset that doesn't lose heart. God is renewing us with every trial and has a lavish celebration awaiting us! Let's make it a point to live our lives in such a way and with such an attitude of grace and thankfulness that people will long to come to the party with us!

Lord God, thank you for today. Thank you for full calendars with lots of people to love in my day, and thank you for empty days with more time to focus on and spend time with you. Thank you for your sacrifice and promise of eternity with you. Help me to be mindful of your plan for me and for those around me in my day. Today is not about me, Lord, but about you! Thank you for giving me a reminder that the stuff of today is temporary. You Lord, are eternal! Amen.

WORKOUT 1 — WEEK 26

WARMUP

3 rounds:

- [ ] 20 lunges (10 each leg)
- [ ] 200-meter run
- [ ] 5 walk-out/walk-ins
- [ ] 20 high skips (10 each leg)
- [ ] 20 jumping jacks
- [ ] 20 arm swings (backward/forward is 1 rep)

WORKOUT

16 minute EMOM:[28]

- [ ] 5 goblet squats
- [ ] 10 jump rope
- [ ] 1 burpee

---

28 "EMOM" stands for "Every minute, on the minute," and means that every time a new minute starts, you do the exercises given. When you've completed them, you rest until the next minute arrives.

WORKOUT 2 — WEEK 26

WARMUP

- [ ] 100-meter jog
- [ ] 10 walk-outs
- [ ] 40 stationary lunges (20 each leg)
- [ ] 30 mock kettlebell swings
- [ ] 15 push-ups
- [ ] 100-meter run

WORKOUT

Complete the following as fast as you can with proper form:

4 rounds:

- [ ] 400-meter run (0.25 miles)
- [ ] 15 kettlebell swings
- [ ] 9 pull-ups (Substitute bent-over dumbbell rows if you don't have a pull-up bar with bands to assist you, or you don't have access to a gym with an assisted pull-up machine.)

WEEK 27

"...and let us consider how to stimulate one another to love and good deeds, not forsaking our own assembling together, as is the habit of some, but encouraging one another..." ~Hebrews 10:24-25, NASB

This past Friday night our box hosted the second workout of the 2013 CrossFit Games Open. In case you're curious and want to give it a go, the workout was a ten minute AMRAP of five shoulder to overheads at seventy-five pounds for females, ten deadlifts (also seventy-five pounds), and fifteen twenty-inch box jumps.[29]

Sometimes I see athletes lying flat on their backs after a tough workout and wonder if they're not just being dramatic, perhaps re-enacting a scene from their favorite war movie. Well, I can tell you that on Friday after my heat ended, I promptly jumped down from the box, and onto my back I went, looking something like a debili-

---

29 "Shoulder-to-overhead" simply means you are to press the weight (in this workout, a loaded barbell) over your head by utilizing a strict press, push-press, or push-jerk. The choice is yours!

tated starfish, I'm sure. Two minutes and a few Lamaze breaths later, I was feeling more alive than ever (props to endorphins)! Everybody did fantastic, and what's more, nobody's shins collided with a box!

After the workout, we all caravanned to a nearby burger place called "Big'z" and camped out at a long picnic table on the patio. As much as I enjoy watching athletes surprise themselves with their ever-increasing strength and newfound abilities during workouts, nothing beats sitting around a table with them as we fuel our bodies with delicious food and our hearts with sharing and laughter.

"A joyful heart makes a cheerful face, but when the heart is sad, the spirit is broken." ~Proverbs 15:13, NASB

The young woman sitting next to me remarked toward the end of the night that her husband (who at present was trying to dissuade those of us ready for a shower and bed from going home at 11 p.m.) is typically a stereotypical homebody by nature.

Perhaps you can relate to this as I can:

Anyway, her husband nodded in agreement before interjecting that on nights like this, being out with a crowd decisively beats staying home on the sofa because "we're out with like-minded people."

This particular "like-minded" bunch of people is fond of spending their Friday evenings sweating hard and cheering loud in a non-air-conditioned gym, followed by hearty eating and merry-making at an open air burger joint. But far more than competing in the Open or talking about how well we did, how far we've come, or how we can improve, the "assembling" of ourselves never fails to transform into an invaluable time of fellowship.

In my experience, "assembling together" in recreational activities with "like-minded" people is often as inspirational as a riveting church sermon and as unifying as a heart-stirring Sunday school class. Every time we engage side by side with others in a workout that leaves us breathless and beaded with sweat, we're conquering mountains and creating memories simultaneously. Reminiscing about the hard parts, reflecting on the victories, and showing off our scars joins us in an unsurpassed symphony of human experience. We become more sympathetic with those training around us. We understand their frustrations, we celebrate in their victories.

Isn't it that way in the Christian's life? Every storm we endure with Christ at the helm and every valley we traverse with the Lord as our Shepherd prepares us to one day be the guiding wind and the soft, sweet light for other afflicted travelers. After the sea has calmed and the peak has been recaptured, we smile and enjoy the view with our friends, those "like-minded" warriors who have faced obstacles, felt pain, fought fear, and found victory through Jesus Christ.

I am so thankful for the body of Christ, his beloved bride for whom he is soon returning. Until he calls us home or sweeps us away to the ultimate banquet (where Paleo and gluten-free are long, lost memories!), we are his ambassadors, his hands and his feet, his eyes and ears, sharing scars, bearing burdens, and breaking bread for his glory.

Dear Gracious God, Steadfast Shepherd of our souls, we thank you for our friends and the love and laughter we receive from fellowship with them. We pray that we will not forsake the assembling of ourselves but instead embrace and enjoy every opportunity we have to gather with our brothers and sisters in Christ. Help us to stimulate one another towards good works and to seek ways to reach out to those who are lost, who need to be a part of a community that loves and serves a living Lord and sanctifying Savior. We pray that Jesus will be at the center of all we say and do today. It is in his name we pray, Amen.

WORKOUT 1 — WEEK 27

WARMUP

2 rounds:

- ☐ 100 jump rope
- ☐ 20 lateral lunges (10 each leg)
- ☐ 20 reverse lunges (10 each leg)
- ☐ 10 walk-out/walk-ins
- ☐ 20 jumping jacks

WORKOUT

20 minute E2MOM:[30]

- ☐ 200-meter run (0.12 miles)

---

30 "E2MOM" means "Every Second Minute, On the Minute," meaning that at the beginning of every other minute, you'll do the given exercise—in this case, you'll run 200 meters.

WORKOUT 2 — WEEK 27

WARMUP

- ☐ 20 lunges (10 each leg)
- ☐ 10 walk-out/walk-ins
- ☐ 20 scorpions (10 each side)
- ☐ 20 high-kicks (10 each leg)
- ☐ 20 reverse lunges (10 each leg)
- ☐ 50 jump rope
- ☐ 10 burpees

WORKOUT

Complete the following as fast as you can, maintaining proper form:

50-30-10 reps of:

- ☐ Air squats
- ☐ Push-ups
- ☐ Double-unders (if unable to do double-unders, sub 150, 90, 30 reps of single jump rope for each set of double-unders, respectively)

WEEK 28

"See to it that no one takes you captive through hollow and deceptive philosophy, which depends on human tradition and the basic principles of this world rather than on Christ." ~Colossians 2:8, NIV

Today, one of the "hollow" and "deceptive" philosophies threatening impressionable young minds and challenging the beliefs of lifelong Christians is *pluralistic universalism*. While I hate to begin a devotional with a text book definition of a hoity-toity word, I think it'll be helpful, so please forgive me!

According to Merriam-Webster, "universalism" is a theological doctrine that all human beings will eventually be saved. You may have heard it put this way: "There are many paths that lead to the same mountain," that mountain being a pleasant afterlife of spectacular sort where we'll all sit together on magic carpets in the clouds plucking our harps, sipping herbal tea, and watching *Friends* reruns. (Okay, so I may have made up a bit of that...)

The Bible warns us that in the latter days, people will follow the false teachings of ungodly teachers who simply preach what carnal, sinful man wants to hear (1 Timothy 4:3). Certainly, it is a warm, fuzzy notion that every last one of us will end up in "the good place," but that couldn't be further from the truth.

Listen to Jesus:

"I am the way and the truth and the life. No one comes to the Father except through me." ~John 14:6, NIV

Christian sister, God sent His only Son to shed every ounce of His blood for *you*. Jesus experienced the most excruciating pain ever endured by a human being at the hands of some of the cruelest tormentors in history. If there had been another way to rescue us from our sins and reconcile us unto God, if we could all ultimately be saved from eternal separation from our Creator regardless of our beliefs, you can be sure God would've spared His Beloved from such unfathomable suffering.

Fit Fact: The word "excruciating" comes from the Latin words "ex" and "cruc" which, put together, mean "from the cross."

Don't be intimidated by the wisdom of today's value system, which is no wisdom at all. When the world tries to make question your faith, remember who you are in Christ. You are a new creation, bought at the extravagant price of Jesus' precious blood (2 Corinthians 5:17). You are more than a conqueror, and nothing—that's right, *nothing!*—can separate you from His love (Romans 8:37, Romans 8:39). You are a child of God and a co-heir of Christ. To put that another way, you are *royalty!* (Romans 8:17).

No one, no matter how many degrees they hold, no matter how many initials are tacked on to their name, can take that away from you. Consider this verse:

The man without the Spirit does not accept the things that come from the Spirit of God, for they are foolishness to him, and he cannot understand them, because they are spiritually discerned (1 Corinthians 2:14).

Pray for those who challenge, even attack you for what you believe. Without the guidance and soul-renewing work of the Holy Spirit in their lives, it will be impossible for them to believe that a Jewish man who died a criminal's death over 2,000 years ago is the only way to Heaven. *With* the Holy Spirit, it is impossible for us to doubt it.

"But examine everything carefully; hold fast to that which is good."
~1 Thessalonians 5:21, NASB

Gracious God, we praise You for sending Your only Son to die for us. Thank You for providing a Way out of the darkness, for lifting the veil from our eyes and teaching us the Truth of salvation. We ask that You would give us confidence, boldness, and grace when we're faced with unsound doctrines that seek to shake our faith. Clothe us with Your armor, secure us with Your strength, and guard our hearts against clever schemes of the evil one who knows his time is short. We pray for our accusers and enemies and ask that You would use us to speak true wisdom into their lives. In the Name above all names we pray, Amen.

WORKOUT 1 — WEEK 28

WARMUP

- [ ] 100-meter jog
- [ ] 20 scorpions (10 each side)
- [ ] 20 butt-kicks (10 each leg)
- [ ] 20 high-knees (10 each leg)
- [ ] 20 squats
- [ ] 200-meter run
- [ ] 10 walk-outs
- [ ] 10 squat-jumps

WORKOUT

14 minute AMRAP:

- [ ] 12 sumo deadlift high-pull with kettlebell
- [ ] 10 alternating kettlebell step-ups onto box (step onto a sturdy bench or table if you don't have a plyo box)
- [ ] 8 sit-ups

AFTERBURN

- [ ] 1-2-3-4-5-6-7-8-9-10 push-ups, resting the same amount of seconds as reps completed (For example, after you do 1 push-up, rest 1 second. After you do the next two push-ups, rest 2 seconds, all the way up to ten.)

WORKOUT 2 — WEEK 28

WARMUP

2 rounds:

- [ ] 20 butt-kicks (10 each leg)
- [ ] 20 high-knees (1o each leg)
- [ ] 20 mountain-climbers (right/left = 1 rep)
- [ ] 15 air squats
- [ ] 15 push-ups
- [ ] 5 burpees

WORKOUT

Complete the following as fast as you can, maintaining proper form:

6 rounds:

- [ ] 6 dumbbell thrusters
- [ ] 200-meter run (0.12 miles)
- [ ] 10 reverse lunges (5 each leg)

AFTERBURN

- [ ] 1-2-3-4-5-6-7-8-9-10 dumbbell bicep curls, resting the same amount of seconds as reps completed (For example, after you do one curl, rest one second. After you do the next two curls, rest two seconds, continuing all the way up to ten.)

WEEK 29

"Join with me in suffering, like a good soldier of Christ Jesus. No one serving as a soldier gets entangled in civilian affairs, but rather tries to please his commanding officer" ~2 Timothy 2:3-4, NIV

Moving beyond being well-trained, physically strong, and fully competent, *good* soldiers are the cream of the crop with more courage than most. They are the ones who perform their duties with all of their hearts, minds, souls, and strength (Luke 10:27). They are the ones who resist the temptation to retreat when the battlefront blazes and the odds stack against them; when their comrades' spirits sink, theirs continue to soar.

This sort of soldier daily dresses himself with the full armor of God:

- Helmet of Salvation
- Breastplate of Righteousness
- Belt of Truth

- Shield of Faith
- Sword of the Spirit
- Shoes of Readiness

Most of those armor pieces are defensive in their design, forged to fight back fiery arrows and thwart deathly blows. It's apparent that this "good soldier" fully intends to see the war out to the end.

While the good soldier is fiercely loyal to his King, he is equally zealous for the men, women, and children who constitute the Kingdom. It's human nature to "look out for Number One" and seek our own fame, wealth, and acclaim, earning badge after badge, moving up the ranks from Private to Sergeant to First Lieutenant. But when we become consumed with the Self and vainglorious aspirations, we are no longer self-sacrificing, which is a chief characteristic of the good soldier:

"Greater love has no one than this, that he lay down his life for his friends." ~John 15:13

In *The Two Towers*, J.R.R. Tolkien wrote:

"War must be, while we defend our lives against a destroyer who would devour all; but I do not love the bright sword for its sharpness, nor the arrow for its swiftness, nor the warrior for his glory. I love only that which they defend."

If I or any "soldier" marching out there loses sight of the "love" which we defend, that is, the name and cause of Christ our Commanding Officer, we're a slow-moving target within the enemy's crosshairs. No longer devoted to the King or receiving the wise orders and counsel of the Commander, it is only a matter of time until our self-made successes, however impressive their impact, come screeching to a halt and our smiles fade at the realization that no amount of money, number of possessions, or multitude of friends can supply true happiness.

I love the Message translation of 1 Timothy 6:6-7:

"A devout life does bring wealth, but it's the rich simplicity of being yourself before God. Since we entered the world penniless and will leave it penniless, if we have bread on the table and shoes on our feet, that's enough."

In this world the air is thick with the intoxicating lures of carnal lust that beckons from billboards and waves from websites, material wealth that shimmers and shines in the media, and the sweet, decadent apple of sin of which we've all partaken. It is only by the strength of the Lord and the daily, conscious act of devoting ourselves to Him that we can be *in* the world but not *of* it, keeping free from the bonds of "civilian affairs" (2 Timothy 2:4).

Dear Lord, our mighty and powerful, patient and kind Commanding Officer, we praise You for giving us another day of life on this earth. And while we fight daily on a spiritual battleground, we know that we are safe beneath Your victorious banner which waves radiantly as a declaration of Christ's finished work on Calvary. Help us to keep our eyes fixed on You, our King, and not to become distracted by the temporary treasures and fading fantasies of this world. We pray to be clothed with Your heavenly armor, fully armed with weapons of faith, truth, righteousness, and salvation. In Jesus' Name we pray, Amen.

WORKOUT 1 — WEEK 29

WARMUP

2 rounds:

- [ ] 20 stationary lunges (10 each leg)
- [ ] 20 high-kicks (10 each leg)
- [ ] 20 stationary butt-kicks (10 each leg)
- [ ] 20 stationary high-knees (10 each leg)
- [ ] 15 air squats
- [ ] 10 push-ups
- [ ] 5 burpees

WORKOUT BENCHMARK WORKOUT

"Perfect Fit Benchmark 1" (Record results in your "Workout Log") and compare your results with Week 15, Workout 1!

16 minute AMRAP (as many rounds as possible):

- [ ] 5 pull-ups (Substitute bent-over dumbbell rows if you don't have a pull-up bar with bands to assist you, or you don't have access to a gym with an assisted pull-up machine.)
- [ ] 7 push-ups
- [ ] 9 air squats

WORKOUT 2 — WEEK 29

WARMUP

2 rounds:

- ☐ 20 reverse lunges (10 each leg)
- ☐ 15 air squats
- ☐ 20 lunges with oblique twist (10 each leg)
- ☐ 10 high skips (5 each side)
- ☐ 10 scorpions (5 each side)

WORKOUT

Complete the following in the order given, maintaining proper form:

- ☐ 50 dumbbell hang-cleans (25 each arm)
- ☐ 50 box jumps (sub 100 squat jumps if you don't have a box)
- ☐ 50 dips

AFTERBURN

- ☐ 60 double-unders for time (sub 180 single-unders if unable to do double-unders)

WEEK 38

"…anyone who competes as an athlete does not receive the victor's crown except by competing according to the rules" ~2 Timothy 2:5, NIV

This week my focus shifts from the metaphor of the courageous soldier to that of the disciplined athlete. Paul writes that in order for any of us to win and be victors of this race—aka, "Life"—we have to abide by the rules…and that takes discipline! In today's *McDonaldized* culture of convenience and quick fixes, easy remedies are both aggressively sold and sought, especially in the areas of health and wellness. Diet pills, exotic *miracle* ingredients, 6-week programs, 7-step plans, machines that melt fat with lipid-seeking Gamma rays…you name it, it's being touted as the latest and greatest fitness tool. "Discipline," in other words, is not a very popular marketing adjective.

This athlete metaphor seems to echo the adage that cheaters never win! If it was my goal to do the 5000-meter run in the Olympics, I wouldn't jog occasionally as training, nor would I fuel my body with cheeseburgers and 7-Eleven Slurpees. To compete on a winning level, athletes daily discipline themselves with strict training, proper diet, and adequate rest.

1 Timothy 4:7 exhorts us to discipline ourselves to be godly. This sort of training is by no means a passive exercise that tolerates a nonchalant attitude or half-hearted effort. There are no shortcuts to godliness and no silver bullets to impede the infernal arrows of the enemy. It is only through an unwavering devotion to prayer and sacred, quiet, *quality* time spent with the Lord that we can truly grow, thrive, and confidently run our race as Christian "athletes."

1 Corinthians 9:24 tells us to run "in such a way as to get the prize." Even though we're not competing against other Christians (there are plenty of crowns to go around in Heaven!), we're still to conduct our lives with the vim, vigor, zeal and zing required of any pro-level athlete.

Charles Simeon was an English clergyman living in Cambridge in the early 1800s when he received a portrait in the mail (photography wasn't around yet). It was a painting of a dear young missionary friend who'd recently died of tuberculosis while serving the Lord in India. After the portrait was unpacked, Simeon couldn't bear to look upon it. Instead he:

"...turned away, covering my face and, in spite of every effort to the contrary, crying aloud with anguish. . . . seeing how much he is worn, I am constrained to call to my relief the thought in Whose service he has worn himself out so much; and this reconciles me to the idea of weakness, of sickness, or even, if God were so to appoint, of death itself. . . . I behold in it all the mind of my beloved brother."

Simeon hung the painting over the fireplace in his living room and in the company of dinner guests would declare, *"There, see that blessed man! What an expression of countenance! No one looks at me as he does; he never takes his eyes off me and seems always to be saying, 'Be serious. Be in earnest. Don't trifle. Don't trifle.'"*

I think those two words best encapsulate the exhortation for the godly athlete. Life is short, a mere mist that appears for a split-second before vanishing into one of two unseen realms, existing in real yet intangible dimensions (James 4:13-14). We have a specific purpose, a unique calling, a specially-designed course mapped out from the beginning (Romans 8:28-30). Let us follow in the on-ward-marching, ever-running footsteps of the soldiers and athletes who've gone before us and were willing to sacrifice all. Let's lean on the Lord to guide us and with His help, never trifle.

Heavenly Father, we praise You for the gifts You've entrusted to us and the races to which you've called us to run with excellence and endurance. We ask for strength to run on any course, in any terrain. No matter the danger, no matter the risks, we know that You make no mistakes, and we can do all things through Your Son who strengthens us (Phil. 4:13). Help us to grow stronger spiritually and physically each day with a Christ-centered commitment to glorify You with our minds, bodies, and souls. In Christ's empowering, eternal name, Amen.

WORKOUT 1 — WEEK 30

WARMUP

3 rounds:

- ☐ 10 reverse lunges (5 each leg)
- ☐ 10 high skips (5 each leg)
- ☐ 10 wall squats
- ☐ 15 mock kettlebell swings

WORKOUT BENCHMARK WORKOUT

"Perfect Fit Benchmark 2" (Record results in your "Workout Log") and compare your results with Week 16, Workout 1!

Complete the following in the order given, with proper form:

- ☐ Timed 1 mile run
- ☐ *Rest* 1 minute
- ☐ 2 minutes: as many sit-ups as possible
- ☐ *Rest* 1 minute
- ☐ 2 minutes: as many air squats as possible
- ☐ *Rest* 1 minute
- ☐ 2 minutes: as many push-ups as possible

WORKOUT 2 — WEEK 30

WARMUP

- [ ] 200-meter jog (0.12 miles)
- [ ] 25 high-kicks
- [ ] 10 walk-outs
- [ ] 25 mock kettlebell swings
- [ ] 15 burpees
- [ ] 200-meter run

WORKOUT

15 minute AMRAP:

- [ ] 20 double-unders (sub 60 single jump ropes if unable to do double-unders)
- [ ] 10 box jumps (sub broad jumps if you don't have a box)

AFTERBURN

- [ ] 3 sets of max plank hold, resting 1 minute between sets.

WEEK 31

"*The hardworking farmer should be the first to receive a share of the crops. Reflect on what I am saying, for the Lord will give you insight into all this*" ~2 Timothy 2:6-7, NIV

Since by now we've mastered what it takes to be both the valiant soldier and the disciplined athlete (note the sarcasm!) we'll move right along to our role as "farmers."

I know nothing about farming; I make weekly visits to warehouse clubs for items necessary for budgeted survival, have thumbs that don't much care for the color green, and skin that has for its sworn enemy that swirling sphere of blazing hot plasma we know as the Sun! But thank goodness the Word of God was written in such a way that even the most agriculturally challenged among us can understand its meaning.

I've observed enough to know (and watched enough movies!) that just like soldiers and athletes, the farmer's work is no walk in the barnyard. He has to prepare and fertilize the soil, plough, sow the seeds, pick the weeds, and finally, reap (I'm sure there are other tasks involved, but researching them would only give me anxiety!). In a figurative sense, I see the farmer as a carefully chosen metaphor representing the Christian's commitment to diligence and resolve to stay the course—or field, as it were—no matter the weather forecast or pesky pasture pillagers.

In order for us to be fulfilled as disciples of Christ living an abundant life here on Earth, effective as ministers, stewards, and servants, and ultimately partakers of His heavenly kingdom, we must first endure the hardship of the harvest, remain steadfast within each season's storms, and stay focused on the ultimate reward: the joyful salvation of our brothers and sisters and the glorious wedding feast at which we will truly taste the goodness of God's bounty.

Throughout your day today, ask the Lord to help you sow seeds where they matter most. Don't burn daylight merely ambling around the perimeter of a perfectly fertile plot of land—get to work and till that ground! Cultivate meaningful relationships. Bear the fruits of the spirit to friends and enemies alike. Give of your crops (gifts and talents, even money, if God leads you) without expecting anything in return. Protect your field from sudden storms and stealthy thieves with continuous prayer and unshakable faith in God's Word.

"Anyone who meets a testing challenge head-on and manages to stick it out is mighty fortunate. For such persons loyally in love with God, the reward is life and more life." ~James 1:12, MSG

Dear Lord, You are fair, and You are just. Your Word tells us that whatever we plant, we will harvest (Galatians 6:7). Let us have the determination and focus of a faithful farmer. We thank You for entrusting to us the tools we need to produce life-giving nourishment to a hurting world. We ask You today to fill us with the strength we need—physically, emotionally, and mentally—to complete today's tasks and endure any hardships that come our way. We know we can do all things through Christ who strengthens us (Philippians 4:13). It is in His Name we pray, Amen.

WORKOUT 1 — WEEK 31

WARMUP

3 rounds:

- [ ] 10 reverse lunges (5 each leg)
- [ ] 10 high skips (5 each leg)
- [ ] 10 wall squats
- [ ] 15 mock kettlebell swings

WORKOUT

10 minute EMOM:

- [ ] 10 kettlebell swings
- [ ] 6 push-ups
- [ ] *Rest* 3 minutes

10 minute EMOM:

- [ ] 4 dumbbell hang-clean each arm
- [ ] 3 burpees

WORKOUT 2 — WEEK 31

WARMUP

2 rounds:

- [ ] 20 butt-kicks (10 each leg)
- [ ] 20 high-knees (1o each leg)
- [ ] 20 mountain-climbers (right/left = 1 rep)
- [ ] 15 air squats
- [ ] 15 push-ups
- [ ] 5 burpees

WORKOUT

Complete the following as fast as you can, maintaining proper form:

- [ ] 16-14-12-9 with 200-meter run between rounds
- [ ] Dumbbell squats
- [ ] Weighted sit-up with dumbbell

AFTERBURN

- [ ] Tabata push-ups

WEEK 32

"Or do you not know that your body is a temple of the Holy Spirit within you, whom you have from God? You are not your own, for you were bought with a price. So glorify God in your body" ~1 Corinthians 6:19-20, ESV

Many of you know by now that one of the monumental verses for my faith-based view of fitness is today's verse above. The Lord used this verse, among others, nearly eight years ago to heal me of the eating disorder that Satan was using to ravage my body and soul (John 10:10). I wanted to share a simple truth that has absolutely freed me from the infernal heaps of condemnation that the enemy launches my direction when I stumble and revert into past sins and struggles: *Repeats of the same spiritual attack are to be expected.*

I've shared publicly that while I *was* healed and I *do* stand victorious in Christ against anorexia and the depression and pride that birthed it, I am not immune to becoming ensnared again. I know from experience and from the testimonials and observance of others that conquering a trial, persevering through a tribulation, or resisting a temptation doesn't drive Satan back to the drawing board where he angrily strikes through the demonic strategies that failed in your life as his soldiers scratch their heads and begin devising a brand new battle plan.

The devil is an old dog with old tricks. And just as he did with Jesus in the wilderness, he'll flee when you resist him, but he'll return after "a season," when "an opportune time" presents itself (James 4:7, Luke 4:13). If he was able to knock you down and draw some blood with a particular dart, don't doubt that he'll select that same arrow from his arsenal again in the future when your defense are down.

"Put on the full armor of God, so that you can take your stand against the devil's schemes." ~Ephesians 6:11, NIV

Stress and idolatry are two hell-sent arrows that come whizzing into my path when verses like 1st Corinthians 6:19-20 become muted in my spirit by the raucous, fruitless efforts of my flesh. When I become anxious and turn to a workout instead of God to clear my head. When I relieve stress by controlling my calorie intake with unhealthy compulsiveness instead of releasing all control to my heavenly Abba—*daddy.* If they endure long enough, these foolish activities lead me down a dangerous, dangerous road…

Just over a year ago, the twin arrows struck me again when a new city, new house, new life as a wife, and then a new business began, well, freaking me out a little bit. I began working out more and ignoring the Holy Spirit and my husband's encouragement to rest, to turn to God, to *be still* (Psalm 46:10). Because I typically lose my appetite when I'm stressed, I was eating less. My temple wasn't being honored at all, but instead, treated like a sheer sack of dust…which it once was before I believed and accepted the redeeming Light of God who sacrificed His life to dwell within it.

From the time of my wedding in December of 2011 to April of last year, my nearly 5'5 frame dropped ten pounds. With the patient and persevering prayers and encouragement of my husband and the Shepherd's strong, steady staff pulling me gently back to His life-giving Word, the arrows have gone up in smoke again, and I am at a healthy weight once more.

Whatever your weaknesses have been in the past, do not be afraid that they will one day overtake you when our age-old opponent finds you vulnerable. Instead, take heart and have hope that your Redeemer has already won the war and is with you this day to fight your battles.

"The LORD will fight for you. Just stay calm." ~Exodus 14:14, NLT

According to the Temple Institute in Jerusalem, the Daily Lotteries at the ancient Temple (destroyed by the Romans in 70 A.D.) decided which priest would be privileged and *honored* that particular day to carry out the important Temple services. All the priests of the family clan who were serving that day would participate in this drawing. This bit of Bible trivia speaks a powerful message to me. You see, those of us who have accepted Jesus as our High Priest have the privilege to tend to the holy temple that He inhabits, our bodies. No daily lottery. No special occasion. It's every day, every hour, every second. What an honor, indeed!

Dear Abba, Father of our glorious High Priest, we praise You for loving us enough to send your Son to die so these sacks of dust we call our bodies could be redeemed, saved from the sting of death, and ultimately glorified in Your heavenly presence one day. We pray that until that day comes, when we need these no more, we will honor them as Your servants once honored the Temple in Jerusalem thousands of years ago. We thank You for the blessing of our health and the tools and knowledge You've given us to wisely care for ourselves and our loved ones. In Jesus' name, Amen.

WORKOUT 1 — WEEK 32

WARMUP

- [ ] 200-meter jog (0.12 miles)
- [ ] 30 lunges with twist over lunging leg (15 each leg)
- [ ] 30 air squats
- [ ] 10 walk-out/walk-ins
- [ ] 30 jumping jacks
- [ ] 15 jump squats
- [ ] 200-meter run (0.12 miles)

WORKOUT BENCHMARK WORKOUT

"Perfect Fit Benchmark 3" (Record results in your "Workout Log") and compare results with Workout 1, Week 18!

Complete the following as fast as you can with proper form:

- [ ] 100 alternating lunges
- [ ] 100 sit-ups
- [ ] 50 push-ups
- [ ] 50 squats

WORKOUT 2 — WEEK 32

WARMUP

- ☐ 800-meter jog (0.5 miles)
- ☐ 10 walk-outs
- ☐ 30 butt-kicks (15 each leg)
- ☐ 30 high-kicks (15 each leg)
- ☐ 30 mock kettlebell swings

WORKOUT

20 minute EMOM:

- ☐ 3 kettlebell swings
- ☐ 3 sumo deadlift high-pulls with kettlebell
- ☐ 3 squat jumps
- ☐ 1 burpee

WEEK 33

"No discipline seems pleasant at the time, but painful. Later on, however, it produces a harvest of righteousness and peace for those who have been trained by it" -Hebrews 12:11, NIV

At the time of this writing, the 2013 CrossFit Open is upon us. Today 100,000 athletes around the world are anxiously awaiting the announcement of the first of five workouts that will be released one at a time for the next five weeks.

At the end of the Open, the top forty-eight men, forty-eight women, and thirty teams from seventeen regions will be invited to compete at the second stage of the CrossFit Games Season, aka, "Regionals."

Granted, only the fittest of the fit will come close to making it to Regionals and then ultimately, to the Games this summer, but every athlete with proven proficiency in the movements is encouraged to participate, no matter their fitness level. Why? Because the Open is an opportunity to accept the challenge to push one's limits. It's a chance to dive into murky waters and leave the crystal-clear comfort of the shallows behind. It's a time to take the strength and skills earned and accumulated over the past year and put them to the test.

Last year was my first time to compete in the Open. The first workout released was seven minutes of burpees. That was it—short, simple, and maybe even sadistic, depending on whom you ask. I performed sixty-four reps in that amount of time while some of the top finishers scored well over one-hundred. At the end of the grueling seven minutes, I had no care that my score was mediocre compared with the rest of the competitors. I gave it everything I had and wanted to pat myself on the back and hang a medal around my neck just for completing it! (If my arms were capable of moving, that is!)

The second workout was a snatch ladder. In ten minutes, the goal was to proceed as far as you could through this sequence:[31]

- 45 pound Snatch, 30 reps
- 75 pound Snatch, 30 reps
- 100 pound Snatch, 30 reps
- 120 pound Snatch, as many reps as possible

I *hated* doing snatches. Probably because I was terrible at them! But for ten minutes, my husband stood close by and coached me through all thirty of the forty-five-pound snatches. I even had four minutes left over to work on fifty, then fifty-five and sixty-pound snatches, all heavier than I'd ever done before. Before the workout began, I was already feeling defeated. Upon finishing, I felt like a conqueror!

The third workout induced even more anxiety for me because it contained a 75-pound push-press as one of its elements, a weight

---

31 The weights shown are those prescribed for female athletes.

which was barely manageable for me at the time. The workout was eighteen minutes of repeating this sequence:

- 15 twenty-inch box jumps
- 12 push-presses
- 9 toes-to-bar[32]

Last year I got ninety-seven reps; I repeated the workout yesterday and PR'ed with 159![33]

I had plenty of excuses (I called them "reasons") not to do the Open last year:

- *I have no aspirations to be a hard-core competitor.*
- *I haven't been doing this long enough.*
- *I'm not strong enough.*
- *I haven't been training hard enough.*

I couldn't be more thankful that despite my catalog of grievances, I participated. I competed…maybe not against the top athletes on the planet, but I competed against my own self-doubt, my complaints, my comfort zone.

And I won.

This week's verse is currently written on the whiteboard at our gym. This verse is true for every discipline in life, from studying for a college exam, waking up at the crack of dawn to work as an unpaid intern, to preparing healthy meals each day and pushing yourself to demolish your doubts, defeat your fears, and erase your excuses in a workout.

---

32 Toes-to-bar are an abdominal exercise in which you hang from the pull-up bar, arms completely extended, and bring your legs upwards until your toes make contact with the bar.

33 "PR" stands for "personal record"

Almighty God, we come to Your throne with thanksgiving and praise, knowing that it is because of Your grace that we can have victory over the fears, trials, and temptations of this life. Thank You for not only guiding us to the challenges and unchartered waters that purify and strengthen us, but also for shepherding us through them. Help us to be like your servant, King David, when he faced Goliath: bold, fearless, fully confident in You, Lord, as His Shield and Sword. We ask for Your strength in Jesus' conquering name, Amen.

WORKOUT 1 — WEEK 33

WARMUP

- [ ] 20 lunges each leg
- [ ] 10 high skips (5 each leg)
- [ ] 20 butt-kicks (10 each leg)
- [ ] 20 high-knees (10 each leg)
- [ ] 200-meter (0.12 mile run)
- [ ] 10 air squats
- [ ] 20 arm circles forward
- [ ] 20 arm circles backwards
- [ ] 10 push-ups

WORKOUT BENCHMARK WORKOUT

"Perfect Fit Benchmark 4" (Record results in your "Workout Log") and compare results with Workout 2, Week 19!

Complete the following three rounds as fast as you can with proper form:

- [ ] 800-meter run (0.5 miles)
- [ ] 15 dumbbell thrusters

WORKOUT 2 — WEEK 33

WARMUP

2 rounds:

- ☐ 20 reverse lunges (10 each leg)
- ☐ 15 air squats
- ☐ 20 lunges with oblique twist (10 each leg)
- ☐ 10 high skips (5 each side)
- ☐ 10 scorpions (5 each side)

WORKOUT

15 minute AMRAP:

- ☐ 5 chin-ups (sub underhanded, bent-over row if you don't have a pull-up bar)
- ☐ 10 burpees

AFTERBURN

- ☐ Tabata calf-raises with dumbbell (alternate legs with each set)

WEEK 34

"Do everything without grumbling..." ~Philippians 2:14, NIV

Last night was CrossFit Open 13.3 at our box. It's been awe-inspiring to stand back and see the powerful truths God is highlighting through this competition, seemingly fashioning it into a fitness buff's parable. From the power of positive words and faith-restoring cheers to the value of camaraderie forged through shared challenges and triumphs, he is showing me just how marvelous, just how matchless, and just how mighty the body of Christ truly is. This week's handwriting on the "wall ball wall" was no exception...

The workout this week was a repeat of last year's 12.4 workout, a twelve minute AMRAP comprised of 150 wall balls, 90 double-unders, and 30 muscle-ups. In twelve minutes, it is the athlete's goal to progress as far through this beastly workout as possible.[34] Some competitors, who I suspect are superhuman vigilantes and cape-wearing world-savers by night, have even managed to begin the sequence for a second time!

I jokingly dubbed this workout "30 Wall Balls" for myself for the simple reason that I, up until yesterday, have included wall balls in my "Top 5 Most-Hated Things List."[35] My bitterness toward the exercise swiftly escalated from a bearable disfavor to full-blown disdain during last year's 12.4, and I can tell you, the transition wasn't pretty.

A fourteen pound medicine ball is an unwieldy object—perhaps more so to me than to others with better coordination—and feeling it crash through my hands and into my chin or chest after every throw was not a pleasurable experience. Standing in my driveway, staring up at a nine-foot-high target of black tape that I was supposed to hit with spot-on accuracy 150 times, I made a decision after twenty sloppy repetitions: "I've had enough. I quit." With the camera still recording and my husband still lovingly encouraging me as my coach and judge to continue trying, I stormed into the house bearing an irreversible hatred for wall balls. Or so I thought…

As soon as 13.3 was announced on Wednesday, I began replaying last year's shameful attempt in my head. I didn't want to feel

---

34 A wall ball is an excellent conditioning exercise in which you stand with a medicine ball 16-24 inches from a wall, perform a front squat, then launch the ball to a target (10 feet above for men, 9 feet above for women) marked on the wall using a push-pressing motion. A muscle-up is a highly advanced gymnastic movement performed on rings suspended from the ceiling in which the athlete uses a forceful kipping, or swinging, motion to propel his or her body over the rings into the bottom of a dip, followed by a press to emerge from the dip.

35 For those curious, my other four Most-Hated Things are snakes, sharks, a host of ubiquitous grammatical errors including, but not limited to, the use of "your" instead of "you're," "alot" instead of "a lot," and "their" instead of "they're," and the temporary cessation of air flow in airplanes before take-off that always makes me question silently if I will ever inhale fresh air again. Oh, and having to turn off my electrical devices before take-off! Okay, that's six, "Six Most-Hated Things."

that frustration again, and frankly, I wanted an excuse not to do it. *I couldn't even get through the first three minutes last year. Fourteen pounds might as well be forty. A nine-foot target might as well be ninety feet. I'm not strong enough. My stamina stinks.* Bah humbug! I thought I had an excuse through my chiropractor. You see, she's been working on the back of my knee for just over a week, using ART (Active Release Techniques) to treat what she suspects is a strained gastrocnemius, a muscle that composes the calf. The back of my knee gives me a mild amount of pain whenever I squat or jump repeatedly. *Maybe attempting 150 wall balls is medically ill-advised,* I thought to myself.

I texted my chiropractor yesterday afternoon. Already aware that I had a rocky relationship with wall balls and excited for me to conquer them, she responded, "Don't be trying to get out of this! You want to come in now?"

Uhhgggg...She's not helping my case at all! I drove to her office where she massaged my leg a bit and adjusted not only my spine, but my attitude. She assured me that my knee would not be exacerbated by performing wall balls, then wrote the following motivational message on the back of my hand:

I love wall balls! I mastered them! I am strong and powerful and unwavering!

How could I not be pumped up after that?! She was right. I was behaving like a "Negative Nancy." I was letting the fear of frustration and one lousy experience prohibit me from even *trying* to prove myself tougher, both mentally and physically, than last year.

This doctor's visit helped cure me of my bad attitude. I completed 13.3 with a score of 127 reps, 107 better than last year, and did so with a smile and a splendid sense of accomplishment. Had I chosen to sit it out, I would've wondered, *What if...?*

I know wall balls are just an exercise, but they've taught me a lesson: *What if?* is the remark of the overcome; *Why not?* is the resolve of the overcomer.

God's gift of life to us is too short to sit on the sidelines, allowing fear, anxiety, doubt, and downbeat attitudes to keep us from victory. We will stumble in this life. We will fall. We will drop the metaphorical medicine ball; the important thing is that we call on God to give us the strength to help us pick it back up again.

Loving Lord, Faithful Father, we thank you for the gift of this life and for the grace you provide for each of its days. Thank you for your unwavering readiness to refill our souls with strength when we feel weak, hope when we feel dismayed, joy when we feel downtrodden, and confidence when we feel inadequate. Help us today to have cheerful, Christ-like attitudes and hearts filled with your Word which assures us of victory through Jesus Christ (1 Corinthians 15:57). Help us to recognize negative thoughts as darts from the enemy and to instantly call upon the truths of Scripture to renew our minds and revitalize our spirits (Romans 12:2). In Jesus' precious name, Amen.

WORKOUT 1 — WEEK 34

WARMUP

3 rounds:

- ☐ 10 high-skips (5 each side)
- ☐ 20 butt-kicks (20 each side)
- ☐ 20 high-knees (20 each side)
- ☐ 100 meter run (0.06 miles)
- ☐ 20 scorpions (10 each side)
- ☐ 10 jump squats

WORKOUT

Complete the following as fast as you can, maintaining proper form:

- ☐ 21-15-9
- ☐ Double-unders (sub 63, 45, 27 single jump ropes if unable to do double-unders)
- ☐ Dips
- ☐ Push-ups

AFTERBURN

- ☐ 5 100-meter sprints (0.06 miles), resting ninety seconds between sprints

WORKOUT 2 — WEEK 34

WARMUP

- ☐ 20 reverse lunges (10 each leg)
- ☐ 50 jump rope
- ☐ 20 high-kicks (10 each leg)
- ☐ 10 lateral lunges (5 each leg)
- ☐ 10 walk-out/walk-ins
- ☐ 10 jump squats
- ☐ 20 mountain-climbers (right/left = 1 rep)

WORKOUT

3 minute AMREP:

- ☐ Dumbbell squats
- ☐ *Rest* 2 minutes

2 minute AMREP:

- ☐ Dumbbell thrusters
- ☐ *Rest* 2 minutes

1 minute AMREP:

- ☐ Burpees

WEEK 35

By	Lezlee Bolcato
Age	27
Occupation	Full-time mom

"And the God of all grace, who called you to his eternal glory in Christ, after you have suffered a little while, will himself restore you and make you strong, firm and steadfast." ~1 Peter 5:10, NIV

A little over two years ago my life was being ripped apart. I had just had my first child and at the same time was ending a toxic relationship. What was supposed to be one of the happiest times in a woman's life was a period of intense chaos and confusion. Even now when I reflect back on those days, I can almost still feel the black wave that was trying to swallow me.

I remember my daily routine was tending to my newborn daughter, and as soon as she would fall asleep I would break down and cry harder than I ever had in my entire life. I didn't understand how I was supposed to be a single parent or how my life had arrived at this place. Nothing could soothe my pain. Not a visit from a good friend, not a family member's supportive words, not food, books, television, nothing.

In my desperation, I turned to the Bible. I had grown up in church and would pray to God, but did not truly understand grace. I went to the back of my Bible and looked up the topic of "suffering." The first verse I chose to read was 1 Peter 5:10. After I read it I immediately felt a peace come over me. For the next few days I read more and more about how we are called to suffer for God. I read how we are supposed to praise Him through our suffering, and that is exactly what I began to do.

At first it felt strange to thank Him when I was having a breakdown, but slowly this lesson began to sink in. I would pray "Thank You, Father, for calling me to suffer. I trust you have a good reason for putting me through this trial. Thank you, Lord, for allowing me to suffer because I know I will boast gladly in Your name knowing that You and You alone have brought me through this storm.

The weeks rolled on and the deeper I dug into His word, the more He revealed His love for me. With His help I began to reclaim my life and discover my identity through Him. When I look at my life now I understand that what happened to me needed to be done in order to regenerate my heart and renew my mind. I am still discovering daily who I am and where He is guiding me.

I look at my life and it's definitely not picture-perfect; it's definitely far from it. I can see the cracks in my character, the shortcomings and pitfalls that distract and derail me, but I no longer try to cover them up. I've learned cover-ups are a shallow way to fix a problem and that the root issue will always resurface. Instead, when I am facing something, I immediately give it to God with the faith that was placed in my heart a couple of years ago. I love the person I am becoming, because with God, I fought to become her.

There are moments that mark your life, and when you are experiencing those tough moments it is hard to believe life will get better. I can promise you it will if you realize that your trials and times of suffering are working to produce steadfastness, like the book of James says. And that steadfastness will one day have its "full effect" so you will be "perfect and complete, lacking in nothing" (James 1:4, ESV). I stumble every day, but I can rest easy knowing I am in His hands and He isn't finished with me yet.

Strengthen us, Father, for we are weak and weary and in constant need of You. Let us know the difference between wanting and needing so we can realize that You alone are all we need. Give us strength to thank You in our weakness so that when we are strengthened again we can exalt Your name. Guide us through our trials. I pray that You will stir in our spirit the faith that we need to know that through difficult times we can call on You. When we face difficult times and it doesn't seem like You hear, help us to go deeper into Your word and faster into Your presence. Let us have the confidence to surrender all to You and rejoice in knowing You have given us these test and trials because You have confidence in our faith to rely on You. I pray for a fullness in our spirit so that all we can do is smile and have the joy of the Lord; we know that the joy of the Lord will be our strength, and that is more than enough for us. In Jesus' name I pray, Amen.

WORKOUT 1 — WEEK 35

WARMUP

- [ ] 200-meter jog (0.12 miles)
- [ ] 30 lunges with twist over lunging leg (15 each leg)
- [ ] 30 air squats
- [ ] 10 walk-out/walk-ins
- [ ] 30 jumping jacks
- [ ] 15 jump squats
- [ ] 200-meter run (0.12 miles)

WORKOUT

Complete the following as fast as you can in the order given, maintaining proper form:

- [ ] 100 sit-ups
- [ ] 90 lunges (45 each leg)
- [ ] 80 air squats
- [ ] 70 push-ups
- [ ] 60 mountain-climbers (right/left is 1 rep)

WORKOUT 2 — WEEK 35

WARMUP

- [ ] 20 lunges (20 each leg)
- [ ] 40 butt-kicks (20 each leg)
- [ ] 20 high-kicks (10 each leg)
- [ ] 20 high-knees (10 each leg)
- [ ] 200-meter run
- [ ] 10 walk-outs
- [ ] 20 forward arm circles
- [ ] 20 backward arm circles
- [ ] 20 jumping jacks

WORKOUT

Complete the following as fast as you can with proper form:

4 rounds:

- [ ] 400-meter run
- [ ] 20 dumbbell push-press

AFTERBURN

- [ ] 1-2-3-4-5-6-7-8-9-10 dumbbell triceps extension, resting the same amount of seconds as reps completed (For example, after you do one extension, rest one second. After you do the next two extensions, rest two seconds, continuing all the way up to ten.)

WEEK 36

By   JoLynn Posey
Age   35
Occupation Stay-at-Home Mom

"So brothers and sisters, since God has shown us great mercy, I beg you to offer your lives as a living sacrifice to him. Your offering must be only for God and pleasing to him, which is the spiritual way for you to worship. Do not be shaped by this world; instead be changed within by a new way of thinking. Then you will be able to decide what God wants for you; you will know what is good and pleasing to him and what is perfect" ~Romans 12:1-2, NCV

It's a new phenomenon for me, but really it's just an old sin manifesting itself in new forms. And I'm learning that the Lord can teach me spiritual lessons just about anywhere.

I'd never been considered athletic until recently, I suppose. I found a groove and discovered a passion for physical fitness. And

I discovered that when I train hard, I feel successful. And when I look good, I feel good. And when I work hard, I can play harder. I'm at times very proud of myself and proud of my changing physique. But I'm discovering subtle layers of sin there, so subtle that these sentiments are praised by just about everybody. But not God. Not in me. Not in this heart that strays off course in the blink of an eye, enticed by something God intended for good, but Satan has warped into wickedness.

The sin didn't start with exercise, nor is the sin inherently exercise itself, but it rears its ugly head here sometimes. The sin is self-idolatry. And I'm guilty.

I'm guilty of choosing a workout over time with the Lord on a busily scheduled day. I'm guilty of spending infinitely more time examining myself in the mirror than I do allowing the Lord to examine my inner self each morning. I'm guilty of pride and boasting after completing a brutal workout. I'm guilty of judging those that choose not to pursue a healthy lifestyle. I'm guilty of centering my thoughts on my physical capacities and appearance rather than on the Lord and His guidance. I'm guilty of expending more time and energy in the pursuit of flat abs than in the fruit of the Spirit. I'm guilty of seeking the praise of others in exchange for giving the praise to the Lord.

Sometimes it just gets out of hand. But I'm growing in the Lord. And I'm beginning to recognize his discipline. I can see how injuries, conflicting schedules, and other obstacles in my workout routine are at times the Lord's intervention. He doesn't want me to continue in my sin, but gently presents opportunity for me to recognize it and repent. He knows that pride and worship of self are much more damaging than a missed workout. I may pay the price of gaining a pound, but I win the reward of shedding the sin.

This isn't a problem simply produced by exercise. This is a sin that is rooted in self-idolatry. When I spend so much time and effort in building myself up, I spend less time exalting the Lord. He alone is worthy of glory. But when I seek praise, glory, and honor for myself, I am creating an idol of myself. I am taking for myself what belongs to the Lord. And I am allowing Satan to take up residence in the Holy Spirit's dwelling place. And once Satan's got a foothold, he's relentless, preying on our very natural sin tendencies. The Lord says that we are the temple of the Living God. As Christians, our bodies actually house the Holy Spirit. And we are to offer our bodies as a living sacrifice to Him. This living sacrifice to the Lord does not equate to a physical sacrifice towards health and beauty. No. Our purpose here is much greater than a long and healthy life. And the prize we strive for is an everlasting crown - far beyond any beauty this earthly body can attain. The Lord created us in his image, to work through us as ambassadors to carry his message to the ends of the earth.

Exercise is not all in vain. I must be ready to answer the call—any call—from the Lord. I want to have the energy and zeal to answer to the Lord's prescription for my day in the same way that I approach the prescribed workout for the day. The products of exercise, such as discipline and endurance, are important in a following-after-Christ lifestyle. We will one day stand before him and give an account as to how we handled the stewardship of this body, our vessels. I want this vessel and its works to be pleasing to Him.

In the offering my body as a daily sacrifice, I must seek to be shaped not by the world—and not by exercise—but to daily seek to be shaped by the Holy Spirit residing in this temple-body. There is a continual renewal of my thinking that must happen as I engage in fellowship with the Holy Spirit in prayer each day. When I'm focused on Him, there's less room for me at the center.

Father God, I love how you love me. I love your gentle leading and your calm discipline. Make my life an offering to you, Lord. Give me each day my daily bread, and give me each day your guidance for my comings and goings that my life may be a fragrant offering unto you. Please convict me of self-worship, for you alone are due all glory. As I seek to be a good steward of this earthly body, may I not lose sight of the prize. Give me a willing heart to sacrifice my will unto yours. In Jesus' precious name I pray, Amen.

WORKOUT 1 — WEEK 36

WARMUP

2 rounds:

- ☐ 20 reverse lunges (10 each leg)
- ☐ 15 air squats
- ☐ 20 lunges with oblique twist (10 each leg)
- ☐ 10 high skips (5 each side)
- ☐ 10 scorpions (5 each side)

WORKOUT

Complete the following as fast as possible, maintaining proper form:

- ☐ 21-18-15-12-9-6-3
- ☐ Burpees
- ☐ Alternating lunges with kettlebell

AFTERBURN

- ☐ Tabata kettlebell oblique twists

WORKOUT 2 — WEEK 36

WARMUP

- ☐ 200-meter jog (0.12 miles)
- ☐ 30 lunges with twist over lunging leg (15 each leg)
- ☐ 30 high-kicks (15 each leg)
- ☐ 10 walk-out/walk-ins
- ☐ 30 jumping jacks
- ☐ 15 jump squats
- ☐ 200-meter run (0.12 miles)

WORKOUT

Complete the following as fast as you can, maintaining proper form:

- ☐ 200 air squats with 10 jump rope On the Minute, Every Minute

WEEK 37

"I know that my redeemer lives and that in the end he will stand on the earth" ~Job 19:25, NIV

Job loved the Lord and had been abundantly blessed with a large family, land, and extraordinary affluence; the dude owned seven-thousand sheep, three-thousand camels, five-hundred yoke of oxen, and five-hundred donkeys. Job 1:3 says he was "the greatest man among all the people of the East."

You've probably heard his story:

Satan—literally, the "Adversary"—is allowed by God Himself to torment Job. This ages-old "Accuser" believes Job will curse God when his health, wealth, and family are destroyed. Despite losing his possessions seemingly overnight—including all ten of his children—and suffering painful boils from head to toe, Job continues to worship and trust God:

"Naked I came out of my mother's womb, and naked shall I return: the Lord has given, and Lord has taken away; blessed be the name of Lord." ~Job 1:20-21, ESV

That's not to say Job didn't cry out in his distress or ask God for reprieve, for just a moment's glimmer in an hour of gloom. In fact, many times Job could not perceive God's presence at all! But Job's faith was so firmly fixed, his spirit so unshakeable, that not one sinful, murmuring word of cursing or complaint ever escaped his lips. He humbly acquiesced to what God had ordained and endured the depths of this world's sorrows with a spirit fully surrendered to following the Father, despite the bleak horizon. After all, he didn't know how his story would end…

The story did end very happily for Job, as it ended happily for Mr. Spafford in yesterday's devotional. Job's health returned, and his wealth was restored with double the number of livestock, seven more sons and three more daughters! (His original ten kids were in Heaven, so that's technically double the children, too!)

But what if Job's story hadn't ended so well? What if he'd died a lonely, diseased, childless widower without a penny to his name? He didn't know all along throughout his suffering that the tide would turn in his favor and that all would be restored. He only knew that the Lord was alive and reigning on the throne. And that was enough.

Is that enough for you? Today, ask yourself how you might respond if everything you worked for and everyone you loved was stripped away. Would you do as Job's wife urged him to do and curse the Lord? Would you become ravaged with guilt and fear, worrying that you'd somehow offended Almighty God? Or would you, like Job, remain faithful, deriving all the strength you need from the simple yet mind-blowing fact that your Redeemer lives, He is unshakable, and all things are in subjection under his feet, even the work of the devil (Ephesians 1:22).

Jesus says it best: *"I have told you these things, so that in me you may have peace. In this world you will have trouble. But take heart! I have overcome the world."* -John 16:33, NIV

Awesome Redeemer, we give thanks that You, and only You, reign in the throne room of Heaven. Your word never returns to You void— your promises are true and eternal (Isaiah 55:11). We thank You that your Word says that nothing—no demon, no depth, not even death—can ever separate us from Your love (Romans 8:38). We ask You to guide us through tribulations, to fill us with your presence so that we can rejoice in all things and turn to you readily, knowing that You possess life-giving water and spirit-sustaining manna. In the Name of Jesus, our Lord and Savior, we pray, Amen.

WORKOUT 1 — WEEK 37

WARMUP

- [ ] 20 butt-kicks (10 each leg)
- [ ] 20 high-knees (10 each leg)
- [ ] 400-meter run (0.25 miles)
- [ ] 10 walk-outs
- [ ] 20 arm circles forward
- [ ] 20 arm circles reverse
- [ ] 20 mountain-climbers (right/left is 1 rep)
- [ ] 20 air squats

WORKOUT

Complete the following as fast as you can with proper form:

- [ ] 100 burpees

WORKOUT 2 — WEEK 37

WARMUP

- [ ] 200-meter jog (0.12 miles)
- [ ] 30 lunges with twist over lunging leg (15 each leg)
- [ ] 20 high-kicks (10 each leg)
- [ ] 20 air squats
- [ ] 10 walk-out/walk-ins
- [ ] 30 jumping jacks
- [ ] 15 jump squats
- [ ] 200-meter run (0.12 miles)

WORKOUT

Complete the following as fast as you can with proper form:

5 rounds:

- [ ] 20 double-unders (sub 60 single jump rope if unable to do double-unders)
- [ ] 15 air squats
- [ ] 10 hand-release push-ups
- [ ] 200-meter run (0.12 miles)

WEEK 38

By   Nicole Babineau

Age   41

Occupation Registered Nurse, wife, mother

"I praise you because I am fearfully and wonderfully made; your works are wonderful, I know that full well" ~Psalm 139:14, NIV

My entire life I have struggled with my weight. I was a chubby child and decided in fifth grade to I wanted to be featured on the *Seventeen Magazine* cover. I began dieting in a healthy fashion and joined "Weight Watchers." I even did Jane Fonda workout videos.

I longed to be perfect. It's a shame I didn't realize then that God saw me that way...

I fell into the enemy's snare and became trapped in an endless pursuit of happiness and fulfillment through weight loss. The diet quickly spiraled out of control, l and by the time I was twelve, I was 82 pounds and hospitalized for anorexia. I spent over a year in the hospital.

I am now forty-two years old and continue to struggle to see myself in a positive light. I struggle to feel "good enough" and satisfied with how I look. I even struggle receiving compliments. I often try to negate it and point out my flaws to the poor person trying to bless me with kind words.

Since October of this year I have been training to run a half-marathon. I have never run one for the simple fact that I really, really do not enjoy running. I have been a member at my CrossFit gym and a Pilates instructor for years, and since running is the one thing I really do not get along with, I am eager to conquer the beast! have faithfully been training since January 1, 2013, adding two short runs during the week and one long run on the weekend to five-days-a-week workout regimen. This is a clear example of overtraining. Not a very smart idea.

Since adding the extra running, I have been riddled with back and hip pain and tight hamstrings. As an athlete, I am accustomed to feeling beat up at times, and I embrace soreness—it means muscles are rebuilding to become stronger. But I have really felt beat down for weeks.

As I was running a few weeks ago, I felt my left calf muscle knot itself into a ball of pain. I had to stop five miles into the run and limp back to the car. I knew before I headed out to the trail that day that my calf wasn't feeling up to running, but I ignored the symptoms and ran anyway. In my head I believed the lie that resting equates to failure and is marker or laziness. "Pain is weakness leaving your body," right?

I recently enjoyed a week off in Disney World on vacation with my husband and two daughters, and as I write it is now the week before the race. I have been praying about whether or not I should run the half-marathon or not. I have asked God to reveal my motivation. I have struggled with the fear of disappointed I signed up to run with. I have heard voices (not literally!) in my head tell me

I'll prove myself to be a loser and a failure if I don't run. They taunt me and say I wouldn't be able to complete the race anyway.

In preparation for Sunday's race, I made an appointment with my massage therapist who is also a close friend. As I lay there on the table confessing my fears to her, it was as if the massage was not only loosening my tight, over-worked muscles, but also unlocking the chains of the enemy.

My masseuse said something to me while I was there that broke me:

"Stop beating yourself up. Be kind to your body."

I thought about this and realized that I have lived my *entire* life abusing the body God gave me. My assignment this week is to rest and recover and take care of this temple.

I've been reflecting on verses such as this one: *"Don't you realize that your body is the temple of the Holy Spirit, who lives in you and was given to you by God? You do not belong to yourself"* (1 Corinthians 6:19).

I don't know if I will run or not. But I *do* know that my worth is not based on whether or not I do. I have decided to consider what God has said about me, that I am his workmanship, created to produce great works that he has already planned for me to do (Ephesians 2:10). That he loves me and chose me (1 Thessalonians 1:4). That I am a saint, and that he is rejoicing over me with joyful songs (1 Corinthians 3:17, Zephaniah 3:17). And there is no condemnation for me in Christ (Romans 8:1).

Lord God, give us eyes to see the beauty in your creation all around us and in ourselves. Thank you that we are fearfully and wonderfully made. Help us to honor you today with our words, actions and bodies. When the enemy draws near, trying to tries to make us doubt who we are and what our purpose is, thank you that your Son is our identity. He is altogether lovely, altogether perfect, and all together wonderful to us. It is in his name we pray, Amen.

WORKOUT 1 — WEEK 38

WARMUP

2 rounds:

- [ ] 200-meter run
- [ ] 10 walk-outs
- [ ] 30 high-kicks (15 each leg)
- [ ] 20 wall squats
- [ ] 50 jump rope

WORKOUT

12 minute AMRAP:

- [ ] 10 suitcase deadlifts with dumbbells
- [ ] 10 alternating step-ups with dumbbells (step onto a sturdy bench or table if you don't have a plyo box)

AFTERBURN

- [ ] Tabata dumbbell walking lunges

WORKOUT 2 — WEEK 38

WARMUP

3 rounds:

- [ ] 10 lunges (5 each leg)
- [ ] 100-meter jog
- [ ] 5 walk-outs
- [ ] 10 high-kicks (5 each leg)
- [ ] 10 butt-kicks (5 each leg)
- [ ] 5 high-knees

WORKOUT

Complete the following as fast as you can, maintaining proper form:

12 rounds:

- [ ] 3 squat-jumps
- [ ] 5 dumbbell thrusters
- [ ] 7 bent-over dumbbell row

WEEK 39

"But put on the Lord Jesus Christ..." ~Romans 13:14, ESV

Browse Pinterest longer than twenty seconds and you're guaranteed to see what other women are "putting on"—or hoping to one day put on—their bodies. From flashy flip-flops and neon running shorts to to vintage jewelry and wedding gowns, the online pin board is a virtual dream-closet, overflowing with the popular designs pinners pine for.

Follow me on Pinterest, and you will find I have pinned to a fashion board a few specific wardrobe items, such as eye-catching sneakers, brightly colored knee-high socks, and sassy sweat bands.[36] Like volleyball players sporting spandex shorts and knee-pads, or cowgirls showing off shiny spurs and bulky buckles, CrossFit

---

36 I'm fond of wearing knee-high socks to protect my shins during deadlifts and box jumps. The extra barrier between the barbell or box and your shins help to reduce the direct friction and will decrease the likelihood of bleeding should you hit the box during a box jump or scrape your leg during a deadlift.

coaches and the athletes we train have our own unique "uniform," if you will. And without saying a word, we tell the world around us what we're passionate about, just by choosing the apparel we "put on." A few weeks ago at a nail salon, for example, I sat next to a woman and immediately noticed she had on a particular brand of shoe that many CrossFit athletes wear. I asked her if she did CrossFit and she nodded with surprise at my accurate assumption. Of course, we proceeded to chat about CrossFit for the duration of our manicures.

From Job *clothing* himself with righteousness in the Old Testament to Paul instructing us to *put on* the full armor of God in the New, God's Word frequently uses the metaphor of dressing ourselves to describe how we are to prepare to walk the Christian walk each day (Job 29:14, Ephesians 6:11). Physical garments cover us, protect us, and yes, express us, and so do spiritual ones. Ever since Adam and Eve with their fig leaves and daily commitment to follow and obey God after being exiled from Eden, every man and woman awakens each morning to clothe themselves both physically *and* spiritually (Genesis 3:7).

I heard Joyce Meyer speak recently on dressing for battle, and she noted quite astutely that "there are certain behaviors that just don't look good on a believer."[37] She explained that just as some colors don't flatter us as well as others, ugly behaviors such as unforgiveness, bitterness, and impatience are unbecoming articles of clothing for a Christian to put on. On the contrary, we look most beautiful, both inside and out, when we don a disposition of compassion, patience, and grace.

Each day, as we put our make-up on for work or our knee socks on for play, let's simultaneously pray to be arrayed with the

---

37 You can listen to Mrs. Meyer's sermon my going to this web address: http://joycemeyer. org/BroadcastHome.aspx?video=Dressed_for_Battle_%E2%80%93_Pt_1

most beautiful Creation in God's grand universe, Jesus Christ himself. Without him, we are naked, exposed to the poisonous darts of the enemy and the carnal caprice of our emotions. Through him, we are clothed with strength when we feel helpless, joy when we feel hopeless, mercy when we feel malicious, thankfulness when we feel envious, and boldness when we feel cowardice. Praise God for the precious gift of Jesus, our Friend, our Savior, our Redeemer, our Refuge!

Abba Father, thank you for this day and all of the blessings and lessons it contains, even for the unknowns that are yet to occur; we trust you with all things because you are Truth and Love. Thank you for your goodness in providing us food to eat, beds to sleep in, and clothes to wear. Help us never to take these blessings for granted, but to give glory to you for every bit of your provision. Lord, we ask today that you would clothe us with your Son so that we may be ready to face any challenge with confidence, accept any praise with humility, and handle any frustration with patience. It is in Jesus' all-sufficient name we pray, Amen.

WORKOUT 1 — WEEK 39

WARMUP

2 rounds:

- ☐ 20 stationary lunges (10 each leg)
- ☐ 20 stationary butt-kicks (10 each leg)
- ☐ 20 stationary high-knees (10 each leg)
- ☐ 20 high-kicks (10 each leg)
- ☐ 15 air squats
- ☐ 10 push-ups
- ☐ 5 burpees

WORKOUT

12 minute ladder:

- ☐ 3 suitcase deadlifts
- ☐ 3 box jumps (sub squat jumps if you don't have a box)
- ☐ 6 suitcase deadlifts
- ☐ 6 box jumps
- ☐ 9 suitcase deadlifts
- ☐ 9 box jumps
- ☐ 12 suitcase deadlifts
- ☐ 12 box jumps

Continue adding three reps to each exercise until 12 minutes are up.

WORKOUT 2 — WEEK 39

WARMUP

2 rounds:

- [ ] 20 butt-kicks (10 each leg)
- [ ] 20 high-knees (1o each leg)
- [ ] 20 mountain-climbers (right/left = 1 rep)
- [ ] 15 air squats
- [ ] 15 push-ups
- [ ] 5 burpees

WORKOUT

Complete the following as fast as you can, maintaining proper form:

- [ ] Run 1 mile, stopping to do 15 air squats at every minute (You'll need a watch for this one!)

AFTERBURN

- [ ] 100 sit-ups for time

WEEK 48

"For momentary, light affliction is producing for us an eternal weight of glory far beyond all comparison" ~2 Corinthians 4:17, NASB

You know by now that the training we're doing is no walk in the park. It's no leisurely jog around your block to the catchy tunes of "Foster the People" or Nicki Minaj. It's no air-conditioned, peppy-paced tour through a state of the art globo gym, gleaming with fancy machinery. It's tough. You sweat. You may even bruise. You push yourself and those around you to keep going, to bound over obstacles and leap over limits, even when it's painful.

Amid the sweat dripping into your eyes, the calluses forming on your palms, and the burning in your muscles, high-intensity training does have one major perk: each session is short—generally speaking, of course! Workouts last, on average, between five and twenty minutes. When I first began, I was pleasantly surprised to find that I could reap such incredible results in so little time. For hours after the workout, I'd enjoy a major endorphin rush—a renewed *joie de vivre*—and my energy levels were sent soaring. No workout ever made me feel so darn good! In just a few weeks, I was already beginning to notice significant improvements in my strength, flexibility, speed, and endurance. I was becoming fitter each day.

All of Paul the Apostle's Christian life was like a gigantic workout, if you will, of the severest nature. Hated for preaching the Gospel, Paul was repeatedly captured and beaten with rods, imprisoned, stoned and left for dead, he was even shipwrecked three times (2 Corinthians 11:25). It's fair to say he endured a substantial bit of discomfort! But to Paul, all of his suffering was merely a "light affliction."

While working out doesn't leave you broken and bleeding on the gym floor (just panting heavily and creating sweat angels upon it at times!) it does qualify as a "light affliction," at least in my opinion. But the weight of the barbells, the height of the box, the distance of the run…all of it produces a "glory" that goes beyond working out to look good in a two-piece swimsuit or burn off Thanksgiving turkey. We bear the physical burdens of dumbbells, kettlebells, medicine balls, and our own bodyweight because doing so makes us stronger and fitter to do the work of the Lord.

It's amazing how much more we can look forward to workouts, however daunting, when our motivation stems from a root of Christ-adoring stewardship and gratitude. Today, let's give thanks for these bodies and their ability to grow stronger, faster, and healthier with each passing day. Let's remember that they are dwelling places of the Holy Spirit and that disciplining ourselves to work out to achieve new goals—new *glories*—ultimately glorifies the One within us.

Dear Lord, thank You for the life-giving truth of Your Word, for the reassuring Scriptures that promise us an everlasting weight of glory, and for all of the tests, trials, and tears that strengthen us until we step into that eternity. Help us to view every storm, whether spiritual or physical, with eyes centered on Your Son and a heart focused on His Kingdom. Show us how to serve You better today with the marvelous bodies You've given us. In Jesus' name, Amen.

WORKOUT 1 — WEEK 48

WARMUP

- [ ] 20 lunges (10 each leg)
- [ ] 10 walk-out/walk-ins
- [ ] 20 scorpions (10 each side)
- [ ] 20 reverse lunges (10 each leg)
- [ ] 50 jump rope
- [ ] 10 burpees

WORKOUT

Complete the following as fast as you can, maintaining proper form:

- [ ] 10-9-8-6-7-5-4-3-2-1 Bent-over dumbbell row, alternated with...
- [ ] 1-2-3-4-5-6-7-8-9-10 decline push-ups (if you don't have a box, you can place feet on the edge of sturdy bench, chair, even a sofa!)

AFTERBURN

- [ ] Tabata superman

WORKOUT 2 — WEEK 48

WARMUP

- ☐ 400-meter jog
- ☐ 10 walk-outs
- ☐ 30 butt-kicks (15 each leg)
- ☐ 30 forward arm circles
- ☐ 30 reverse arm circles
- ☐ 20 arm swings (backward/forward is 1 rep)
- ☐ 20 jumping jacks

WORKOUT

Complete the following as fast as you can in the order given, maintaining proper form:

- ☐ 100-meter run (0.06 miles)
- ☐ 25 goblet squats with kettlebell
- ☐ 200-meter run (0.12 miles)
- ☐ 15 goblet squats with kettlebell
- ☐ 400-meter run (0.25 miles)
- ☐ 5 goblet squats with kettlebell

AFTERBURN

- ☐ Tabata burpees

WEEK 41

"If God be for us, who can be against us?" ~Romans 8:31, KJV

This world is full of things that come against us: diseases, unhealthy hormones in our food, pollutants, the economy, natural disasters, evildoers, satanic attacks, even our own friends and family, to name a few. It's easy to get discouraged in this fallen, sin-cursed world. Even when we're certain God has called us to a particular job or endeavor, it's easy to think, *How can I ever succeed at this?*

The early church is a powerful example of assured victory with Christ, even in the face of ferocious persecution. Christians in the Roman Empire were viewed as a despicable, criminal people. Emperor Nero went so far as to blame them for the fires that swept through Rome in 64 A.D. and consequently threw them to wild beasts or burned them alive as human torches.

Twenty-five years later under Emperor Domitian, Christians ironically were deemed "atheists" and therefore were considered "dangerous to human civilization" (*Roman History,* Dio Cassius).

Many scholars believe the Apostle John, who penned the last book of the Bible, "Revelation," was exiled during his reign.

That a once tiny sect of Judaism could grow to become the world's dominant religion despite centuries of continuous persecution testifies to God's steadfast promise to prosper and protect His people and plans. We can be certain that our hands will succeed at whatever task the Lord has placed them on, no matter the might and magnitude of our opposition.

Today, remember that the same Holy Spirit that raised Christ from the grave and emboldened the early church to stand firmly by the Word of God and empowered them to preach, serve, and heal is the One who dwells in you! Don't let the enemy or words from the world steal your joy or make you question your commitment to God's purposes in your life. He will always reward you for your faithfulness.

*"And without faith it is impossible to please him, for whoever would draw near to God must believe that he exists and that he rewards those who seek him." ~*Hebrews 11:6, ESV

Blessed Father, we live in a frightening place. Each day brings with it bad news and countless threats that, if we let them, could rid us completely of our peace. Lord, we thank You for sending Your Son to us who promised to be with us always, even to the end of the age (Matthew 28:20). Help us to know that no weapon formed against us will prosper because You are greater than any evil, seen or unseen (Isaiah 54:17). We ask this in the eternally strong, eternally powerful Name of Jesus, Amen.

WORKOUT 1 — WEEK 41

WARMUP

- ☐ 30 lunges (15 each leg)
- ☐ 20 butt-kicks (10 each side)
- ☐ 20 high-knees (10 each side)
- ☐ 20 mountain-climbers (right/left is 1 rep)
- ☐ 20 reverse lunges (10 each leg)
- ☐ 10 broad jumps

WORKOUT

Complete the following as fast as you can, maintaining proper form:

5 rounds:

- ☐ 30 air squats
- ☐ 20 push-ups
- ☐ 10 burpees

WORKOUT 2 — WEEK 41

WARMUP

- ☐ 400-meter jog (0.25 miles)
- ☐ 20 lunges (10 each leg)
- ☐ 20 scorpions (10 each side)
- ☐ 20 high-kicks
- ☐ 20 reverse lunges (20 each leg)
- ☐ 20 mock kettlebell swings

WORKOUT

10 minute AMRAP:

- ☐ 200-meter run
- ☐ 20 kettlebell swings

AFTERBURN

- ☐ 3x max wall-sits

WEEK 42

By	Andrea Tabler
Age	49
Occupation	Women's Ministry Coordinator and owner of marketing and graphic design firm

But he said to me, 'My grace is enough for you. When you are weak, my power is made perfect in you.' So I am very happy to brag about my weaknesses. Then Christ's power can live in me. For this reason I am happy when I have weaknesses, insults, hard times, sufferings, and all kinds of troubles for Christ. Because when I am weak, then I am truly strong" ~2 Corinthians 12:9-10, NCV

Pursuit of perfection. It's the subtle temptation the enemy whispers into my ears each day. After all, why not strive for perfection? Certainly there's nothing wrong with a clean and thoughtfully decorated home with a well-manicured yard (just don't open any cupboards or, even worse, peek in the garage). Our yearly Christmas card shows my family's smiling faces on our most recent beach vacation (when, in fact, we may have weathered a difficult family crisis that year). I show up to church appearing "put together" in my favorite new outfit from J. Crew (the outlet store, lest you think I'm a frivolous spender), when all morning I've obsessed over the fact that I've put on four pounds in three months. *This* is where the enemy has his most fun with me.

If I'm honest, I must admit that I spend much of my time pursuing perfection in all I do in every area of my life. But this manifests itself the most when it comes to my physical appearance perfectionism…my body image. I know in the quiet places of my soul that I was fearfully and wonderfully made, created and chosen by my loving Father God. But when I put on my favorite jeans and they feel snug, I'm sent into a tailspin, longing—no, desperate—to fix the "problem." Because of my distractions and my focus on the trivial and the earthly, I completely miss out on the special plans and delights Jesus has set before me that day.

My Lord tells me not to be anxious about anything, especially my body. But time and time again I ignore His words and find myself in an endless cycle of thought processes that don't lead to the abundant life he has promised me. When I'm caught up in the rat race of physical perfectionism, fueled by the unrelenting desire to fit back into my way-too-snug white pants, I eat healthy and faithfully (no, neurotically) exercise on a daily basis. Once the pants have adequate wiggle room, I'm lured back to brie cheese, Jelly Bellies and pizza, and my fitness goals are forgotten.

Yet daily, the lover of my soul calls to me, wooing me back into his presence. When I choose to listen, he draws me close to him, and I leave the pursuit of perfection and success behind. I am nourished by his life-giving Word…by his *love*. I walk (run, and do burpees) in confidence, whether or not my tummy jiggles in the process. Because my confidence is in him. He lovingly reminds me that his grace truly is sufficient for me.

But how do I consistently *dwell* in that grace place, conquering the enemy's attempts to kill, steal and destroy by dangling the quest for perfection before me each morning when I step on the scale? How do I manage to listen to the voice of Truth rather than the father of lies? Only in community with other believers who encourage me, admonish me and "do" life with me. Working out with my sisters in Christ has become one of those communities for me. A place where there's no makeup or trendy clothes but instead an environment where we can be real and vulnerable—despite our imperfections—and seek God's best for us together. With these sisters, I press forward to conquer that next workout that my flesh says is impossible. We cheer each other on and text messages of encouragement, prayers and scripture. Through this loving community, Jesus reminds me that this fragile, weak, and broken girl is made strong in him alone. I don't need perfection. I just need Jesus.

Father God, thank you for loving me even when I stray into the sinful territory of perfectionism. Thank you for reminding me you made me just the way YOU wanted. Thank you for my precious sisters in Christ that you use in amazing ways in my life. And thank you for your grace that is all sufficient at every turn of my life. I ask for your forgiveness for the times I loathe this body—this temple—you lovingly created. I accept that only in my weakness am I truly strong in you, so I can stop the crazy quest for perfection! I pray this in Jesus' holy name. Amen.

WORKOUT 1 — WEEK 42

WARMUP

- ☐ 100-meter jog
- ☐ 20 scorpions (10 each side)
- ☐ 20 butt-kicks (10 each leg)
- ☐ 20 high-knees (10 each leg)
- ☐ 20 squats
- ☐ 200-meter run
- ☐ 10 walk-outs
- ☐ 20 forward arm circles
- ☐ 20 reverse arm circles

WORKOUT

Complete the following as fast as you can, maintaining proper form:

21-15-9:

- ☐ Dumbbell hang-cleans each arm
- ☐ Squat jumps

AFTERBURN

- ☐ Run 400 meters (0.25 miles) for time.

WORKOUT 2 — WEEK 42

WARMUP

2 rounds:

- [ ] 20 reverse lunges (10 each leg)
- [ ] 15 air squats
- [ ] 20 lunges with oblique twist (10 each leg)
- [ ] 10 high skips (5 each side)
- [ ] 10 scorpions (5 each side)
- [ ] 10 mock kettlebell swings

WORKOUT

Complete the following as fast as you can with proper form:

3 rounds:

- [ ] 15 kettlebell swings
- [ ] 18 chin-ups (sub underhand bent-over dumbbell row if you don't have a pull-up bar)
- [ ] 21 sit-ups

WEEK 43

"Let us run with endurance the race God has set before us" -Hebrews 12:1, NKJV

"Hey! CrossFit 925 works!!! 5:06 marathon, which is one minute faster than my old record. And I did it only by working out at the gym —no runs! ...It's a great feeling to run a marathon without spending all your spare time on the road running—boring..."

That was a text I received one Sunday afternoon from Stefan, one of our incredible coaches at CrossFit 925. Stefan has been a competitive marathoner and triathlete for some time, so the completion of this marathon wasn't a milestone, per se. What *is* remarkable about this particular achievement is that it was accomplished without adhering to a strict marathon training regimen.

All Stefan did to prepare is what myself, my husband, and the people we coach at the box do four to five times a week, on average, and that's high-intensity, constantly varied workouts.

Many of our athletes have been flabbergasted by their athletic improvements, not only in strength and flexibility, but in endurance, speed, and stamina as well.[38] People who have never been able to run a mile in their lives are doing so now…and enjoying it! Others' mile times decrease with almost every attempt. The funny thing is, we don't run one whole mile at once very often, and yet everything else we do undoubtedly—if not mysteriously—trains us to be, among other things, strong runners.

This marathon-prepping, mile time-improving "phenomenon" (for lack of a better word), brings to mind our spiritual race, one that calls for marathon-like commitment, discipline, focus, and endurance.

The road of the Christ-follower is not only narrow, it is fraught with peril, pain, and persecution (Matthew 7:13). The moment we "sign up" to run this race, the devil pins a target on our backs, and it flaps in the wind all of our lives like a black and white bib number. As marathon runners are plagued by bad weather, blisters, shin splints, and sprains, the race of the Christian is paved with countless obstacles that seek to derail and immobilize us (John 10:10). And if you've been on this planet long enough, you know that some obstacles are much larger than others…

A failed exam. A fender bender on the way home from work. A fight with your spouse. An argument with your best friend. These commonplace trials are 5-Ks and fifteen-minute workouts in comparison to the marathon-sized events—such as the sudden death of a loved one, the heart-wrenching throb of divorce, the bleak cold words of a cancer diagnosis—that truly test our faith, try our patience, and show our strength.

James, the brother of Jesus, wrote 2,000 years ago, that trials and tests produce perseverance (James 1:3). Every struggle in life,

---

38 We everyone who does CrossFit is considered an "athlete," by the way! Our motto at CrossFit 925 is "Discover Your Inner Athlete."

no matter the size, is significant. Every frustration, every discouragement, every mistake holds value because each one has the power to make us stronger, more prepared, and better equipped to face the hardships ahead. These gentler paths through winter's wind give us strength for summer's gale.

Stefan wasn't aware that every workout was preparing him for his fastest marathon yet, but he can look back today at how wondrously the deadlifts, the squats, the box jumps and burpees trained him for the rigors of a five hour, six minute marathon. Whatever we've been through, let us "consider it pure joy," joy to fuel us for the marathon (James 1:2). And above all, let us never forget that we are ultimately striving for a crown that never perishes at the end of that finish line.

Father in Heaven, how great Thou art! How immeasurable Your love for us, how innumerable the wonderful future You have planned for us! How unworthy are we to deserve and inherit even one iota of the good that flows from Your throne! And yet, by the cross of Christ, we are made co-heirs with Your Son and will be rulers in Your kingdom, all because Yours is a throne of grace (Romans 8:17, 2 Timothy 2:12, Hebrews 4:16). Help us take the trials in our lives, the struggles, the tears, the disappointments, and surrender them to You to purify and strengthen us for the storms ahead. We know that You work all things together for good, even the things that seek to depress, discourage, and destroy (Romans 8:28). Help us always keep the ultimate finish line at the forefront of our minds so that we can run with untiring endurance the race You've mapped out for us. In Jesus' enduring name, Amen.

WORKOUT 1 — WEEK 43

WARMUP

2 rounds:

- [ ] 20 stationary lunges (10 each leg)
- [ ] 20 high-kicks (10 each leg)
- [ ] 20 stationary butt-kicks (10 each leg)
- [ ] 20 stationary high-knees (10 each leg)
- [ ] 15 air squats
- [ ] 10 push-ups
- [ ] 5 burpees

WORKOUT BENCHMARK WORKOUT

"Perfect Fit Benchmark 1" (Record results in your "Workout Log") and compare your results with Week 29, Workout 1!

16 minute AMRAP (as many rounds as possible):

- [ ] 5 pull-ups (Substitute bent-over dumbbell rows if you don't have a pull-up bar with bands to assist you, or you don't have access to a gym with an assisted pull-up machine.)
- [ ] 7 push-ups
- [ ] 9 air squats

WORKOUT 2 — WEEK 43

WARMUP

- [ ] 20 lunges (10 each leg)
- [ ] 10 walk-out/walk-ins
- [ ] 20 scorpions (10 each side)
- [ ] 20 reverse lunges (10 each leg)
- [ ] 50 jump rope

WORKOUT

- [ ] In 6 minutes, complete 60 sit-ups as fast as you can and then complete as many burpees as possible.

AFTERBURN

- [ ] Tabata reverse lunges

WEEK 44

"In peace I will lie down and sleep, for you alone, O LORD, will keep me safe" ~Psalm 4:8, NLT

How well did you sleep last night? Did slumber come swiftly, soon after your head hit the pillow, or were worries and questions from the day blazing boisterously through your mind, forbidding sweet dreams from ever approaching, even chasing away the sheep as you began to count?

According to the U.S. Department of Health and Human Services, approximately 60 million Americans suffer from insomnia each year. The Mayo Clinic's website defines insomnia as "a disorder that can make it hard to fall asleep, hard to stay asleep, or both." A number of things can cause insomnia, such as stress and anxiety, depression, or Seasonal Affective Disorder (SAD). And for those of us who are able to fall asleep normally, we often don't get *enough* sleep. A study from the National Sleep Foundation found that 20 percent of Americans reported getting only six hours of sleep or less each night in 2009, two hours shy of the recommended amount of eight hours.

Why all this chatter about snoozing? Because it's extremely important! Just look at the harms that accompany sleep deprivation:[39]

- Increased risk of motor-vehicle accidents.
- Increase in body mass index (BMI) due to an increased appetite caused by sleep deprivation.
- Increased risk of diabetes and heart problems.
- Increased risk for psychiatric conditions including depression and substance abuse.
- And a decreased ability to pay attention, react to signals or remember new information.
- Just as an improper diet negatively impacts our waking functions, inadequate sleep dreadfully affects our daily lives as well, preventing us from feeling our best and giving our all to our various jobs and duties as sisters, wives, daughters, friends, students, and workers, in whatever capacity.

As you might guess, given our previous devotion about God's care and concern for the foods we eat, our Father is equally interested in seeing to it that His children are sleeping soundly, peacefully, every night of the week.

King David had more reason than us all, I'd dare say, to be a restless sleeper. He had battled and slain a giant as a boy, was fiercely hated and hunted by the jealous King Saul, and then as king of Israel, committed adultery with a married woman and had her husband killed, a sin which precipitated a curse upon his own family, leading to the death of his newborn son. Another son, Amnon, raped his own half-sister and was killed by another brother, Absalom. Absalom then led a revolt against his father and was

---

39 http://www.foxnews.com/health/2011/02/25/sleep-really-need/#ixzz2DGsdZ5Ou (accessed November 12, 2013)

ultimately defeated and killed by David's troops. I think it goes without saying that David had more than his fair share of stressful situations, heartaches and hardships.

And yet, David's hand penned today's verse: *"In peace I will lie down and sleep, for you alone, O LORD, will keep me safe."* How could a man with so many enemies and so much tragedy sleep so soundly? Because he left the big things—his safety, his throne, his very life—in God's hands. Despite his sins and his failures, he knew that God's love would never abandon him.

No matter the sins we've committed, no matter the size of the burden we feel bearing down on us, no matter the hole left in our hearts after the death of a loved one, God is still on His throne. And His eyes are still on you. While you are sleeping, He's holding the stars and moon in place and appointing angels to stand guard for all His children (Psalm 91:11). You can sleep well knowing that you are ever in your Father's thoughts and in His vision.

Dear Holy Father, we thank You for our wonderfully made bodies, bodies that were marvelously designed, destined to serve and perform myriad assignments, meant to experience countless joys and pleasures, all for your glory. We pray that You would help us to rest soundly in the knowledge of Your sovereignty, knowing without a doubt that You are always in control and hold all things together (Colossians 1:17). Thank You for Your precious Son Jesus, who was able to sleep in the midst of a terrifying storm, providing the ultimate example of what it looks like to trust and place our faith in You alone (Matthew 8:24). In His Name we pray, Amen.

WORKOUT 1 — WEEK 44

WARMUP

3 rounds:

- ☐ 10 reverse lunges (5 each leg)
- ☐ 10 high skips (5 each leg)
- ☐ 10 wall squats
- ☐ 15 mock kettlebell swings

WORKOUT BENCHMARK WORKOUT

"Perfect Fit Benchmark 2" (Record results in your "Workout Log") and compare your results with Week 30, Workout 1!

Complete the following in the order given, with proper form:

- ☐ Timed 1 mile run
- ☐ *Rest* 1 minute
- ☐ 2 minutes: as many sit-ups as possible
- ☐ *Rest* 1 minute
- ☐ 2 minutes: as many air squats as possible
- ☐ *Rest* 1 minute
- ☐ 2 minutes: as many push-ups as possible

WORKOUT 2 — WEEK 44

WARMUP

- [ ] 20 reverse lunges (10 each leg)
- [ ] 50 jump rope
- [ ] 20 high-kicks (10 each leg)
- [ ] 10 lateral lunges (5 each leg)
- [ ] 10 walk-out/walk-ins
- [ ] 10 jump squats
- [ ] 20 mountain-climbers (right/left = 1 rep)

WORKOUT

Complete the following as fast as you can, maintaining proper form:

4 rounds:

- [ ] 8 dumbbell clean and jerk, right arm
- [ ] 10 suitcase deadlifts
- [ ] 8 dumbbell clean and jerk, left arm

AFTERBURN

- [ ] 1-2-3-4-5-6-7-8-9-10 dips, resting the same amount of seconds as reps completed (For example, after you do one dip, *rest* one second. After you do the next two dips, *rest* two seconds, continuing all the way up to ten.)

WEEK 45

By	Ashley Donde
Age	29
Occupation	PR for Documentary Film Production Company and Mommy of 2

"Therefore, whether you eat or drink, or whatever you do, do all to the glory of God" ~1 Corinthians 10:31, NKJV

When I joined my CrossFit gym in June 2012 I fell in love instantly, like many of you. Seeing myself do things I never thought I'd do, building camaraderie with my friends at the gym, feeling healthy and happy, and, as a mother of 2 young children, having some "me" time at the end of my day all kept me coming back for more.

That ended abruptly after only three months of training when a pull-up bar snapped during a workout and came crashing down on my head, splitting it open and resulting in 6 staples and a mild traumatic brain injury. I fell into a deep depression, was unable to work out in any capacity for 4 months, and went through what were basically the stages of grieving. It. Was. Awful.

When I started coming back in January 2013, it was incredibly hard to see the friends I had invited to the gym lifting heavier, getting double-unders, and kipping while I was basically starting all over. Talk about discouraging! All I wanted to do was go back in time and change what had happened. Accepting my reality was a hard pill to swallow, and my own pride made it even harder.

I share this because we so often compare ourselves with each other, as Christians and as athletes. I often finish last in a workout due to my slow recovery and want to tell everyone "I'm still recovering, that's why it takes me so long!" I hate being last. I hate thinking anyone at my box thinks I'm "out of shape" or "lazy." As followers of Jesus we are "recovering" from our sin nature. We won't be perfected until we reach heaven. Sometimes that "recovery" seems slow at times as well, especially if we compare ourselves to each other.

Pride is such a nasty trait. When we're the first one done in a workout and gloating in our success, or the last one done thinking, "I'm too good to be the last one to finish!" the root of the thought is still the same: it's all about ME. When I'm at the gym and it's all about "me" I will be endlessly frustrated and never satisfied. There will ALWAYS be someone better. I will probably get some kind of injury again (hopefully just some minor setback next time!), illness, etc. that will keep me from being one-hundred percent for a time. I need to learn this pride lesson NOW. Jesus needs to be the satisfaction of my soul. HE is all I need, and everything else He gives me to enjoy is just a bonus! We must be careful not to turn our pleasures into vices. The same goes for my walk with Christ. It's not about how "Christian" I look compared to my friends. It's about me and Jesus. It's that simple.

I love the story of Olympic runner Eric Liddel (portrayed in the film *Chariots of Fire*). He used his gift of running for the glory of God and said, "When I run I feel His pleasure." Ok ladies, how awesome is that?! May we feel God's pleasure as we glorify him with our bodies. Throw out the pride, and be filled with His Spirit. Don't compare your Christianity or your fitness to anyone else's. You belong to Jesus. Do it all for Him!

Lord, forgive us for our pride—for seeing ourselves as better than others—and not reflecting the humility of Christ. Help us to find our security in your son, Jesus. May all our satisfaction in life, all our pleasure come from your hands. May we reflect the beauty of our loving and selfless Savior back into this fallen world as we daily die to our flesh. And may all we do be for your glory. In the name of Jesus we pray, Amen.

WORKOUT 1 — WEEK 45

WARMUP

- ☐ 20 lunges each leg
- ☐ 10 high skips (5 each leg)
- ☐ 20 butt-kicks (10 each leg)
- ☐ 20 high-knees (10 each leg)
- ☐ 200-meter (0.12 mile run)
- ☐ 10 air squats
- ☐ 20 arm circles forward
- ☐ 20 arm circles backwards
- ☐ 10 push-ups

WORKOUT

12 minute AMRAP:

- ☐ 200-meter run (0.12 miles)
- ☐ 20 overhead walking lunges with dumbbells (10 each leg)
- ☐ 30 double-unders (sub 90 single jump ropes if unable to do double-unders)

WORKOUT 2 — WEEK 45

WARMUP

- ☐ 400-meter jog
- ☐ 10 walk-outs
- ☐ 20 arm circles forward
- ☐ 20 arm circles reverse
- ☐ 20 mountain-climbers (right/left is 1 rep)
- ☐ 20 air squats
- ☐ 5 jump squats

WORKOUT

6 minute EMOM:

- ☐ 3 dumbbell squats
- ☐ 3 hand-release push-ups
- ☐ 3 box jumps (sub broad jumps if you don't have a plyo box)
- ☐ *Rest* 3 minutes

6 minute EMOM:

- ☐ 6 pull-ups (sub bent-over dumbbell row if you don't have a pull-up bar)
- ☐ 2 burpee/box jumps (sub burpee/broad jump if you don't have a plyo box)

WEEK 46

"And we know that God causes everything to work together for the good of those who love God and are called according to his purpose for them"
~Romans 8:28, NLT

> *Though Satan should buffet, though trials should come,*
> *Let this blest assurance control,*
> *That Christ has regarded my helpless estate,*
> *And hath shed His own blood for my soul.*

Those are some of the lyrics to one of my favorite hymns, "It Is Well with My Soul."

You may have heard about the harrowing circumstances surrounding the song's composition. I'll give you the Spark Notes version:

The hymnist, Horatio Spafford, was an attorney living in Chicago in 1871 when the Great Fire swept through the city, nearly destroying everything he owned. Just one year prior, his only son had died of scarlet fever at the age of four.

In 1873, Spafford planned a European holiday with his family which would coincide with one of Moody's meetings being held in England (like a Billy Graham crusade, I would imagine). Due to an unexpected business delay, Spafford stayed behind in Chicago a while longer and sent his wife and four young daughters ahead of him to France.

Tragically, their steamship was struck by an iron sailing vessel, and two-hundred twenty-six lives were lost, including those of his daughters. His wife Anna was spared her children's fate simply -and yet, profoundly -because a wooden plank floated beneath her unconscious body and held her above the waves. She heard a disembodied voice speak, "You were spared for a purpose."

It was while sailing back across the Atlantic, having viewed the very place where his daughters had perished, that Spafford was inspired to pen what has become one of the most enduring and beloved hymns, especially for those surrounded, struggling, or immersed in their own dark sea of sorrow, grief, anguish, and travail.

The story ended happily for the Spaffords. They bore three more children, and despite losing yet another young son to illness, they continued to faithfully serve the Lord.

And as for that "purpose" Anna's life was spared to fulfill, she and her husband followed a call to settle in Jerusalem where they founded the "American Colony" with a mission to show and share Christ's love by serving destitute, outcast, and ailing people, no matter their religious affiliation or ethnicity.

The couple's ministry throughout orphanages, hospitals, soup kitchens, and other charitable institutions continues to this day in Jerusalem with the name, the Spafford Children's Center. It is a well-respected, highly venerated outreach in the Holy City that serves over 30,000 Jewish and Arab children each year. Talk about "legacy!"

"It's easy to be grateful and good when you have so much, but take care that you are not a fair-weather friend to God."
~words recalled by Anna Spafford

No matter what you're going through, whether a deep dark forest of thorns and thieves or an open sea of still blue waters and a heavenly breeze, know that the Lord has a plan, a perfect plan. Trust only in Him and you will find immense happiness on the other side of your heartache, breathtaking beauty beneath your brokenness.

Gracious God, we lift up Your holy Name with hearts awestruck by Your unending mercy and eternal love that overflows. We thank You for your unchanging faithfulness and the immutable promises of Your Word, promises that include taking the disappointments, failures, tragedies, and tears of our lives and using them to mold for us a future that is surer, stronger, brighter than anything we could have imagined. Help us to lean on You, our Captain, our King, in every kind of weather. In Jesus' Name, Amen.

WORKOUT 1 — WEEK 46

WARMUP

- ☐ 200-meter jog (0.12 miles)
- ☐ 30 lunges with twist over lunging leg (15 each leg)
- ☐ 30 air squats
- ☐ 10 walk-out/walk-ins
- ☐ 30 jumping jacks
- ☐ 15 jump squats
- ☐ 200-meter run (0.12 miles)

WORKOUT BENCHMARK WORKOUT

"Perfect Fit Benchmark 3" (Record results in your "Workout Log") and compare results with Workout 1, Week 32!

Complete the following as fast as you can with proper form:

- ☐ 100 alternating lunges
- ☐ 100 sit-ups
- ☐ 50 push-ups
- ☐ 50 squats

WORKOUT 2 — WEEK 46

WARMUP

3 rounds:

☐ 10 reverse lunges (5 each leg)
☐ 10 high skips (5 each leg)
☐ 10 wall squats
☐ 15 mock kettlebell swings

WORKOUT

Complete the following as fast as you can, maintaining proper form:

☐ 100 kettlebell swings with 1 burpee on the minute, every minute

WEEK 47

By	Erica Shimamura
Age	30
Occupation	Client support specialist at CrossFit Bandera Road

"Therefore put on the full armor of God, so that when the day of evil comes, you may be able to stand your ground, and after you have done everything, to stand. Stand firm then, with the belt of truth buckled around your waist, with the breastplate of righteousness in place, and with your feet fitted with the readiness that comes from the gospel of peace. ~Ephesians 6:13-15, NIV

I began this fitness journey when I abruptly came to a crossroads. With no family to cling to and my mother's suicide leaving me broken and bitter, I felt lost at sea.

My emotions were everywhere and all-engulfing. The entire universe seemed to overwhelm me for what felt like a lifetime. I had some amazing people in my life and some not-so-amazing. I was partying non-stop and abusing my body with bad food, drugs, and alcohol. I was tired all the time. I was desperate for something else, to feel rested and at peace. My parents had nothing, and when I lost them, I felt I had even less than nothing. I remember my mother always telling me about God and his goodness and love, but had ignored her wisdom much of my adult life. Out of sheer desperation I began to attend Bandera Road City Church and found myself healing and recovering.

It was there, overcome with despair, that I begged on my knees for a sign, for mercy from this addiction and this affliction of loneliness. I tried to understand why would God take everything away from me and keep me here on this earth weak, tired, and alone. It was then I began to see the Lord and how he'd been keeping me safe even in my darkest hours. I found my way, this path to God's goodness—he had cleared it for me.

I found my "God-time" in my training. I learned that every individual's daily routine needs a quiet space, a space that's just between us and God, a space to listen to his guidance. I have been in sadness, felt hopelessness, and been on my knees begging for God's mercy in compromising situations I knew I had no control over. I was paralyzed by my weak spirit and had allowed clouds of pessimism to overcome me. I began to find that a stronger body was building a stronger mind, and that created the bridge to a better life.

I began to feel stronger for having completed something, to have chosen to do a list ("workout") of challenging—some would say torturous—deeds that made me feel stronger; and not just stronger for me, but also for others who need someone to help them keep going.

I realize now that I have a choice. I choose this temporary pain for the ultimate gain. I remind myself of the victim I once was, the victim on her knees begging for strength. I remind myself of what it felt like to be humbled by the burning in my muscles and remembering that out in the world there are countless others feeling that way, and not just about AMRAP or "5 Rounds for Time," but about their lives seemingly crumbling before them. It is humbling. It softens my heart, and God speaks to me as I remember...

I am grateful for the choice of victory over victimization. Because of it, I am becoming a stronger, healthier individual. Not because I want to be hot stuff in a bikini, but because I truly aim to invest in becoming strong from the inside out and to be strong for this world I live in. When I am out of breath and on my knees, looking to the skies for an answer, I remember how good it feels to have the strength to stand up and help others, help them fight to regain their hope and joy.

I am blessed to be able to share the Gospel through my testimony and through CrossFit Bandera Road. Whatever your past is, God will use it to teach and strengthen you for your future. Your life is a beautiful journey, and the Lord is with you to make it through, conquering all the way.

Dear Lord, help us to be strong in faith and spirit, to trust in your glory and divinity. Help us to lean on you and know unequivocally that even in our despair and darkness, you will carry us through and through, to the light of a new day. We know that the armor we need comes from the Spirit you sent to dwell within us, and the desires of our hearts will be manifested when we delight in you. In the name of your Son we pray to be beacons of light in a dark world, courageous fighters on Satan's battlefield, peacemakers in a volatile society, peacekeepers in our families and relationships, and above all, lovers of Christ, Amen.

WORKOUT 1 — WEEK 47

WARMUP

- [ ] 20 lunges each leg
- [ ] 10 high skips (5 each leg)
- [ ] 20 butt-kicks (10 each leg)
- [ ] 20 high-knees (10 each leg)
- [ ] 200-meter (0.12 mile run)
- [ ] 10 air squats
- [ ] 20 arm circles forward
- [ ] 20 arm circles backwards
- [ ] 10 push-ups

WORKOUT BENCHMARK WORKOUT

"Perfect Fit Benchmark 4" (Record results in your "Workout Log") and compare results with Workout 1, Week 33!

Complete the following three rounds as fast as you can with proper form:

- [ ] 800-meter run (0.5 miles)
- [ ] 15 dumbbell thrusters

WORKOUT 2 — WEEK 47

WARMUP

- ☐ 400-meter jog
- ☐ 20 high-knees
- ☐ 20 butt-kicks
- ☐ 20 sit-ups
- ☐ 20 scorpions
- ☐ 20 mock kettlebell swings

WORKOUT

15 minute AMRAP:

- ☐ 100-meter run (0.06 miles)
- ☐ 10 weighted sit-ups with dumbbell
- ☐ 10 Russian kettlebell swings each arm

AFTERBURN

- ☐ 50 superman for time

WEEK 48

By Merrily Mann-Brown

Age: 50

Occupation: Marketing Consultant

"Where there is no vision, the people perish…" ~Proverbs 29:18, KJV

Have you had days when you struggle to get out of bed, because you just lack the zeal, the motivation, or the energy? Perhaps you have days where you get out of bed only because of habit or obligation, but you face the day feeling rather bored.

I used to feel those days more often than not. I dreaded to face another mundane day filled with mediocre routines. I was going through life without much purpose. I lived each day without much intention. I certainly wasn't a "winner."

I would drag through the day, pulling with me the weight of past mistakes, regrets, and shame.

I went to a Christian Business Women's Luncheon last year. We started out in prayer, asking God to reveal to us our purpose and to instill in us his dream for our lives.

Then they asked us close our eyes and picture our dream or our vision, only go bigger. And then go bigger, and then go bigger.... They had us picture what we looked like, how we felt, and a few other things I can't remember at the moment.

What was interesting is I didn't picture myself overweight and out of shape. I didn't picture myself sitting in front of the television with a bowl of popcorn-heavy-on-the-butter. I didn't picture myself sitting at a bar downing margaritas. I didn't picture myself lying in bed. And I wasn't sad or depressed.

I pictured myself comfortable in my non-plus-sized clothes, I was happy, I was energetic, and my hair looked pretty. My house was clean and my office was tidy. My dishes were done and my bed was made.

After the luncheon, I went home and deleted most of my shows on the DVR. I know...strange first step! Sitting in front of the TV suddenly seemed like a waste of time. The next day I went to my first class at CrossFit 925.

Since that day eight months ago, I've been exercising three to five days per week. I've read more books than I have in the last five years. I've connected with some awesome women. I've made my bed every morning. I've lost several pants sizes. I really feel I'm headed in the direction of the vision that God gave me.

Eight months ago I was lazy, fat, and always tired. I had to drag myself out of bed. Today I'm full of energy and excited about tomorrow. It all started with vision.

So what does it take to "win?" One of my favorite sayings from years back is: *You can't shoot a target you can't see.* Make sure you ask God for his vision for your life. Once you see that vision, make sure that everything you have or do in your life aims you in the right direction for that vision. Discipline will come much easier when you take the right aim. Determination (or passion) will come as well.

Dear Father God, I ask that you help me see clearly the vision you have for my life. Burn it into my heart so that I can come alive with the passion and excitement that Your vision can bring. Help me to take the steps that clearly lead to your promises fulfilled. Some days I drag, God. Some days I feel bored. Some days I feel weak. Let your Holy Spirit fill me. Help me to overflow with your passion, your love, and your direction. I want to bring you Glory, God. Amen.

WORKOUT 1 — WEEK 48

WARMUP

2 rounds:

- [ ] 20 reverse lunges (10 each leg)
- [ ] 15 air squats
- [ ] 20 lunges with oblique twist (10 each leg)
- [ ] 10 high skips (5 each side)
- [ ] 10 scorpions (5 each side)

WORKOUT

Complete the following as fast as you can with proper form:

3 rounds:

- [ ] 50 air squats
- [ ] 7 pull-ups (sub bent-over dumbbell rows if you don't have a pull-up bar)
- [ ] 14 dips
- [ ] 21 push-ups

WORKOUT 2 — WEEK 48

WARMUP

3 rounds:

- [ ] 10 reverse lunges (5 each leg)
- [ ] 10 high skips (5 each leg)
- [ ] 20 high-kicks (10 each leg)
- [ ] 10 wall squats
- [ ] 15 get-ups

WORKOUT

18 minute AMRAP:

- [ ] 10 Turkish get-ups with dumbbell (5 each arm)
- [ ] 400-meter run (0.25 miles)

WEEK 49

By	Ann Marie Dillashaw
Age	41
Occupation	Stay-at-home mom and homeschool teacher

"Fear not, little flock, for it is your Father's good pleasure to give you the kingdom. Sell your possessions, and give to the needy. Provide yourselves with moneybags that do not grow old, with a treasure in the heavens that does not fail, where no thief approaches and no moth destroys. For where your treasure is, there will your heart be also" -Luke 12:32, ESV

I am thankful that The Lord was pleased to allow my journey to cross paths with the love of a CrossFit coach and friend. Each day at the box, information is shared, like the number of push-ups, push-presses, or air squats we'll be doing—oh how I hate air squats—and instructions are given, like how to do a power snatch correctly or a pull-up more efficiently. And almost every day, I read and hear stories of battles lost and victories won concerning a heart that is tempted to treasure food more than God.

The same sorts of workout programming and personal testimonies are shared in gyms all across the world. The difference for me is the revelation of a loving heavenly Father guiding me on a journey to find satisfaction in Him alone, to glorify Him in all that I do.

Just like a workout description on paper cannot cause the fat to fall off my body, the mere knowledge that Jesus loves me is not a useful weapon against an enemy that seeks to kill, steal, and destroy (John 10:10). The treasure acquired along the journey is far lovelier and more valuable than anything I ever gained from information alone.

This revelation has brought meaning to life that helps me, on most days, reject the offering of unhealthy or excessive amounts of food and laziness. This revelation strengthens me to seek the greater treasure of disciplining my body for the glory of God. This revelation allows me to forget the shame of battles lost to diets that do not work and instead seek the treasure found in a lifestyle that desires a healthy body to fight the good fight of faith.

The Word breathes life into a body that was headed down a path of spiritual shambles and physical death, while giving me a love for people to help them do the same. The journey to trust in the Father's good pleasure empowers me to no longer treasure insignificant calories from fatty foods, but to glorify Him in the hard places of a workout.

I pray that today the eyes of your heart are opened to your journey. That information turns from knowledge to a believing faith rooted in love. That your journey leads to the defeat of shame and guilt and soldiers on toward life abundant in Jesus.

Father God, help your children to hear the sweet words of Jesus, "Blessed are you...for flesh and blood did not reveal this to you, but my Father who lives in Heaven" (Matthew 16:17). Let these words empower us to seek to glorify your name in all we do. In your sweet Son's name we pray, Amen.

WORKOUT 1 — WEEK 49

WARMUP

2 rounds:

- [ ] 20 lunges (10 each leg)
- [ ] 20 high kicks (10 each leg)
- [ ] 5 walk-out/walk-ins
- [ ] 20 high-knees (10 each leg)
- [ ] 20 butt-kicks (10 each leg)
- [ ] 50 jump rope

WORKOUT

Complete the following as fast as you can in the order given, maintaining proper form:

- [ ] 30 burpees
- [ ] 800-meter run (0.5 miles)
- [ ] 20 broad jumps
- [ ] 400-meter run (0.25 miles)
- [ ] 10 burpee-broad jumps
- [ ] 200-meter run (0.12 miles)

WORKOUT 2 — WEEK 49

WARMUP

3 rounds:

- [ ] 10 high-skips (5 each side)
- [ ] 20 butt-kicks (20 each side)
- [ ] 20 high-knees (20 each side)
- [ ] 100 meter run (0.06 miles)
- [ ] 20 scorpions (10 each side)
- [ ] 10 jump squats

WORKOUT

Complete the following as fast as you can, maintaining proper form:

5 rounds:

- [ ] 15 kettlebell swings
- [ ] 20 dumbbell lunges (10 each leg)
- [ ] 100 jump rope

WEEK 50

"You will eat the fruit of your labor; blessings and prosperity will be yours" ~Psalm 128:2, NIV

Ever since Adam and Eve ate the forbidden fruit offered to them in Eden, even the godliest men and women have labored to earn honest wages, build stable, respectable lives, and raise God-fearing children, all by the sweat of their brows (Genesis 3:16-19).

"Labor" is defined in the Merriam-Webster dictionary as an "expenditure of physical or mental effort especially when difficult or compulsory." There's a good reason "labor" is synonymous with "childbirth" and why a national holiday, aptly deemed "Labor Day," honors those who sacrifice and devote long hours to both contribute to society and strengthen our economy. Labor is, well, *laborious.*

Even though Adam and Eve's sin contaminated creation with the toils of the "nine-to-five" and the distresses of carrying and delivering a child, God graciously kept intact a promise of blessing and prosperity to those who work diligently. So while work, whether in a job or in the home, is often stressful, exhausting, and at times, nearly impossible, we can rejoice in the midst of it knowing that rest and rewards are reserved for the faithful.

After coaching athletes through exceptionally challenging workouts, I often ask, "So, how do you feel?" I can't recall a single time when one of them has responded with a negative or remorseful answer. After they've caught their breath and sipped some water, they reply with exclamations such as these:

"I feel awesome!" and, *"I'm so proud of myself! I didn't think I could do it, and I did!"*

Some even go so far as to say they want to do the formerly "killer" workout again soon! (In those instances, I suspect it's just the endorphins talking.)

The next time they enter the box and see a formidable-looking workout scrolled across the whiteboard, they think twice before labeling it "Impossible!" Why? Because they've proven to themselves that they're stronger than they think. They've proven that hard work yields blessings of confidence, of strength, of happiness and greater health. They know that if they authoritatively rid their minds of worry, boldly replace all fears with faith, and courageously *labor* to conquer the day's challenge, they *will* be victorious.

"...overwhelming victory is ours through Christ, who loved us" ~Romans 8:37, NLT

In life and in fitness, with our families and with our workout communities, giving one-hundred percent of ourselves is never a wasted effort. When we strive to honor God by working willingly and wholeheartedly at everything we do as Colossians 3:23 instructs, the fruit we'll receive will be sweet, full of life-giving nourishment for mind, body, and soul, and we will soon catch our breaths, sip some water and say, *"I feel awesome!"*

Whatever challenge presents itself today, whatever workout (whether in this book or elsewhere!) makes you perspire just looking at it, remember that victory, sweeter than any Red Delicious the enemy could offer, is waiting for you to bite into it if you would simply trust in Jesus to be your strength.

"The LORD is my strength and my shield; my heart trusts in him, and he helps me." ~Psalm 28:7, NIV

Dear Abba, Father, Giver or sweet rewards, Keeper of blessed promises, thank you for this day and all the splendor it holds, including the beauty of shadowy valleys, murky waters, even frightening workouts. We know you make all things beautiful and pray that you would stir within us the courage and willingness to see each challenge through to its radiant end, where blessings and prosperity are reserved for us. We thank you for your Son, without whom we can no nothing. We thank you for your Spirit who helps us to bear your supernatural fruit, like joy, peace, patience, and faithfulness. Help us to honor you in every task in every hour of every day. In Christ's name we pray, Amen.

WORKOUT 1 — WEEK 50

WARMUP

- ☐ 30 lunges with twist over lunging leg (15 each leg)
- ☐ 30 air squats
- ☐ 10 walk-out/walk-ins
- ☐ 30 jumping jacks
- ☐ 15 jump squats
- ☐ 400-meter run (0.25 miles)

WORKOUT

Complete the following as fast as you can, maintaining proper form:

10-9-8-7-6-5 alternating between:

- ☐ Dumbbell thrusters
- ☐ Push-ups
- ☐ *Rest* 3 minutes

5-6-7-8-9-10 alternating between:

- ☐ Double-unders (sub 15-18-21-24-27-30 singe jump ropes if unable to do double-unders)
- ☐ Push-ups

WORKOUT 2 — WEEK 50

WARMUP

2 rounds:

- [ ] 20 butt-kicks (10 each leg)
- [ ] 20 high-knees (1o each leg)
- [ ] 20 mountain-climbers (right/left = 1 rep)
- [ ] 15 air squats
- [ ] 15 push-ups
- [ ] 5 burpees

WORKOUT

Complete the following as fast as you can, maintaining proper form:

- [ ] 400-meter run, then:
- [ ] 21-15-9
- [ ] Pull-ups (sub bent-over dumbbell row if you don't have a bar)
- [ ] Oblique twists with dumbbell
- [ ] 400-meter run

WEEK 51

"Everything that lives and moves will be food for you. Just as I gave you the green plants, I now give you everything" ~Genesis 9:3, NIV

We live in amazing times. We have access to the world through just a few clicks of our fingers across a keyboard. Through websites and corresponding video and photos, we can virtually travel anywhere we choose. At the same time, we can flip on the TV and eavesdrop on the daily drama of strangers' lives via a "reality" show, or listen to news anchors report on an earthquake shaking the west coast, a bomb scare in the Middle East, even a happy tale of a puppy finding its way home somewhere in your city. We can transport ourselves miles and miles to a movie theater or mall in under an hour by hopping in a little innovation called a car.

After building an appetite exploring the world either vicariously through the Internet or literally through modern transportation, we can prepare food in just minutes using modern appliances, such as a blender or a microwave oven. If still out and about, we can opt to remain in our cars and order drive-through at a nearby fast food restaurant! (Yuck!)

In this incredible age of convenience, it's easy to forgo healthy, God-made foods in favor of man-made, processed junk foods that do more harm than good. Today's verse states clearly that our food should come from sources that live and move (well, at least they *used to*!). Refined and processed foods such as corn syrup, cookies, crackers, white rice, and canned fruits and vegetables.

Refined foods are nutritionally imbalanced, stripped of important vitamins and minerals. The food God has planted are grown in orchards, greenhouses or gardens, are unprocessed and unrefined, and have a shorter shelf life. These foods are naturally flavorful, have gorgeous colors, and appetizing textures. Moreover, they are full of the micronutrient vitamins, minerals, antioxidants, phytochemicals, and fiber.

God didn't just give us plants to eat, but animals as well (for a full list of God-approved critters, check out Leviticus 11 and Deuteronomy 14). But not just any turkey leg or bison burger will do; make sure it's as close to its original state as possible. We put ourselves at an increased risk for certain cancers when we consume processed meats. Turkey cuts found at the deli counter, for example, contain nitrates, which are shown to be carcinogenic.

Try to buy certified organic meats as often as you can to avoid the laundry list of artificial ingredients and chemicals attached to the labels of the processed stuff. Remember, fueling your body with the proper nutrients that God intended for it not only guarantees a happier, healthier life, it glorifies our Maker!

Dear Lord, Maker of Heaven and Earth and everything in them, we thank You for all You've so graciously provided for us, from the air we breathe, the talents you've given, to the roof over our heads and food on our tables. We pray that You would give us the knowledge, discipline, and discernment to eat the foods that our bodies respond to best, food that fuels us with life-giving nutrients so we can better serve You and others around us. Thank You for the fruit on the trees, the vegetables in the ground, the fish in the sea and cows in the pastures. Most of all, we thank You for the Bread of Life, Your Only Son who gave His life for us. In His Name we pray, Amen.

WORKOUT 1 — WEEK 51

WARMUP

3 rounds:

- [ ] 10 high-skips (5 each side)
- [ ] 20 butt-kicks (20 each side)
- [ ] 20 high-knees (20 each side)
- [ ] 100 meter run (0.06 miles)
- [ ] 20 forward arm circles
- [ ] 20 reverse arm circles
- [ ] 10 jump squats

WORKOUT

Complete the following as fast as you can, maintaining proper form:

8 minute AMRAP:

- [ ] 8 dumbbell push-press
- [ ] 12 box jumps (sub squat-jumps if you don't have a plyo box)

AFTERBURN

- [ ] Tabata tricep push-ups

WORKOUT 2 — WEEK 51

WARMUP

2 rounds:

- [ ] 20 reverse lunges (10 each leg)
- [ ] 15 air squats
- [ ] 20 lunges with oblique twist (10 each leg)
- [ ] 10 high skips (5 each side)
- [ ] 10 scorpions (5 each side)

WORKOUT

Complete the following in the order given as fast as you can with proper form:

- [ ] 50 air squats
- [ ] 50 push-ups
- [ ] 50 lunges (25 each leg)
- [ ] 50 renegade rows (25 each arm)
- [ ] 50 goblet squats
- [ ] 50 sit-ups
- [ ] 50 dumbbell suitcase deadlifts
- [ ] 50 double-unders (sub 150 single jump ropes if unable to do double-unders)

WEEK 52

"God, the one and only— I'll wait as long as he says. Everything I need comes from him, so why not? He's solid rock under my feet, breathing room for my soul, An impregnable castle: I'm set for life" ~Psalm 62:1-2, MSG

Our CrossFit box is currently hosting an eight-week challenge called "Skinny Santa" this year in which participants weigh in and record their weight and body fat percentage once a week. More than anything, we're hoping to motivate our athletes to stay on track during the eight-week-long pig-out fest into which the holidays so easily morph. But sometimes I just want to say *to the North Pole!* with the scale where it can be imprisoned in an icy igloo of shame and guilt alongside the Grinch, Scrooge, Lucy van Pelt, and other nefarious Christmas villains.

One of the ladies I coach recently had a revelation regarding her "on again/off again" relationship with the scale.

She once weighed over 400 pounds. After having a gastrectomy, altering her diet, and committing to a consistent workout schedule, she was just a few pounds away from reaching the 200 Pounds Lost milestone. Anticipating this achievement began to consume her, pushing her to weigh in daily so she'd be certain to catch the winning numbers smiling up at her like a triumphant slot machine. But the day she expected that number to show up, it wasn't there.

She stepped onto the scale religiously for days, only to watch the numbers increase one pound, then two pounds, all adding up to one incalculable word: FRUSTRATION. Last week when the other "Skinny Santas" were taking off their socks, hoodies, and all other "bulking" materials in preparation for the weekly weigh-in, she wisely declined. Like a ubiquitous Taylor Swift love song, she was breaking up with the scale. For a while, at least.

Like so many of us, she had allowed the quiet power of the scale to become Dictator of her mood, Discourager of her progress, Destroyer of her joy, and a Distraction from her ultimate goal to glorify God as she pursues physical fitness for His kingdom. Let's not let what could be a helpful tool become a harmful idol in our lives. This woman's lesson should be a lesson for all of us in that it reminds us that it is *God* who is our Source, our Strength…in *everything*. He's the One enabling us to be successful, to have victory, and we will continue to be conquerors as long as we keep our eyes fixed on Christ and His perfect purpose for our lives. The moment we let our eyes fall to the sparkling lures of the world and follow them like fish down a broad, meandering stream is the instant we let those things rule us.

"Don't love the world's ways. Don't love the world's goods. Love of the world squeezes out love for the Father. Practically everything that goes on in the world—wanting your own way, wanting everything for yourself, wanting to appear important—

has nothing to do with the Father. It just isolates you from him. The world and all its wanting, wanting, wanting is on the way out—but whoever does what God wants is set for eternity." ~1 John 2:15-17, MSG

Dear Lord, Giver of Life and Destroyer of Death, we thank You for hardwiring into our beings an inextricable desire to wonder and to worship, to gaze up at the stars and ask Who made them so we can adore their Maker. We pray that You would help us keep our eyes looking to You and our hearts pining to bow at Your feet. Keep us from temptation, including the temptation to fixate on and idolize objects, such as food, the gym, the tape measure, or the scale. Help us to remember that You alone are our Ultimate Strength and our Way to complete health and victory in all matters in life, and that when we seek You first, You will surely provide us with all good things (Matthew 6:33).

WORKOUT 1 — WEEK 52

WARMUP

- ☐ 100-meter jog
- ☐ 20 scorpions (10 each side)
- ☐ 20 butt-kicks (10 each leg)
- ☐ 20 high-knees (10 each leg)
- ☐ 20 mock kettlebell swings
- ☐ 200-meter run
- ☐ 10 walk-outs
- ☐ 20 forward arm circles
- ☐ 20 reverse arm circles

WORKOUT

14 minute AMRAP:

- ☐ 400-meter run (0.25 miles)
- ☐ 14 alternating Russian kettlebell swings (7 each arm)

AFTERBURN

- ☐ 50 kettlebell swings for time

WORKOUT 2 — WEEK 52

WARMUP

- ☐ 200-meter run
- ☐ 20 high-kicks (10 each leg)
- ☐ 20 air squats
- ☐ 30 lunges with oblique twist (15 each side)
- ☐ 10 squat jumps
- ☐ 30 mock kettlebell swings
- ☐ 10 push-ups

WORKOUT

Complete the following as fast as you can, maintaining proper form:

4 rounds:

- ☐ 10 alternating kettlebell step-ups onto box (step onto a sturdy bench or table if you don't have a plyo box)
- ☐ 15 burpees
- ☐ 20 walking lunges with kettlebell (10 each leg)

AFTERBURN

- ☐ Tabata oblique twists with kettlebell

APPENDIX A
THE EXERCISES

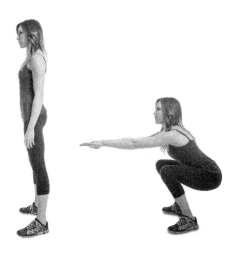

AIR SQUAT

A. Stand with your feet spread apart at a distance slightly wider than the shoulders. Position your feet so that your toes angle out. This angle varies from person to person, but should be about 30 degrees. Keep your weight on the heels to prevent yourself from rolling up onto the balls of your feet.

B. Keep your chest up, shoulders back, head up. This helps promote a nice, safe, intact lumbar curve.

C. Place arms straight out in front of your chest. The arms should be in a comfortable position as they act as counter balance to the motion of the exercise.

D. Bend your knees as you lower yourself down. Pretend there is a chair behind you that you're reaching back to sit on. Your knees should track over your feet and never jut out over them. In other words, your knees should be pointing in the same direction as your toes. If you find your knees starting to cave in, focus on pushing them out. A good way to achieve this is by imagining you are tearing the floor apart with your feet.

E. The push back up should be generated from your hamstrings and glutes. Your chest and head should remain pointing straight forward. As you rise, your arms will probably lower back to your sides naturally. Make sure your knees keep tracking with your toes and do not begin to buckle inwards. Also be sure and keep your lumbar curve intact (curved). Generally speaking, if you have your chest and head up, your lumbar curve will be in the correct position.

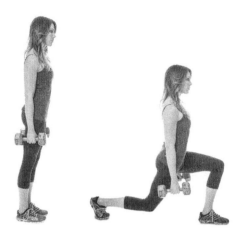

ALTERNATING DUMBBELL LUNGES

A. Stand with feet shoulder-width apart, torso upright with arms hanging straight at your sides with a dumbbell in each hand.

B. Take a slow, controlled lunge forward with one foot, keeping arms straight. As you lunge, lower your body and allow the lunging knee to bend until your thigh is parallel to the ground.

C. Push explosively off the lunging foot to return to the starting position.

NOTE: Make sure your torso stays upright. Do not lean forward toward the dumbbells as you lunge.

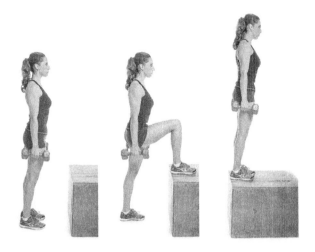

ALTERNATING DUMBBELL STEP-UP ONTO BOX

A. Stand behind a plyometric box (18 to 20 inches tall) with dumbbell in each hand.

B. Place one foot on the box and push through your heel to stand on top of it.

C. Straighten your leg completely before bringing your other foot (trailing leg) on top.

D. To finish, step down with the trailing leg, keeping your body weight shifted on the lead leg.

E. Repeat with the opposite leg leading and repeat for the given number of repetitions.

NOTE: Make sure you don't drop onto the trailing leg on your descent.

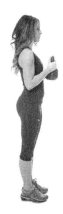
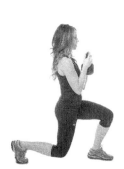

ALTERNATING KETTLEBELL LUNGES

A. Hold a kettlebell by its horns at your chest. Stand with feet shoulder-width apart, torso upright.

B. Take a slow, controlled lunge forward with one foot, keeping the kettlebell close to your chest. As you lunge, lower your body and allow the lunging knee to bend until your thigh is parallel to the ground.

C. Push explosively off the lunging foot to return to the starting position.

NOTE: Make sure your torso stays upright. Do not lean forward toward the dumbbells as you lunge.

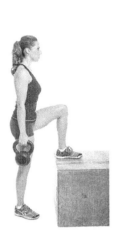
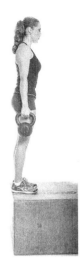

ALTERNATING KETTLEBELL STEP-UP ONTO BOX

A. Stand behind a plyo box (18 to 20 inches tall) with a kettlebell in one hand.

B. Place the opposite foot as hand holding kettlebell on the box and push through your heel to stand on top of it.

C. Straighten your leg completely before bringing your other foot (trailing leg) on top.

D. To finish, step down with the trailing leg, keeping your body weight shifted on the lead leg.

E. Switch the kettlebell to the other hand and repeat with the opposite leg leading. Repeat for the given number of repetitions.

NOTE: Make sure you don't drop onto the trailing leg on your descent.

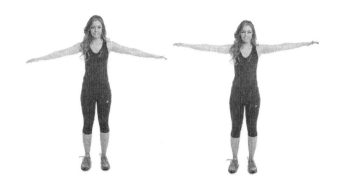

ARM CIRCLES
(FORWARD AND BACKWARD)

A. Stand in a neutral position with feet hip-width apart. Your arms should be straight out to the sides so your body forms a "T."

B. Begin making slow circles in a forward motion with your arms, then gradually make larger ones and complete the given number of repetitions.

C. Repeat in the opposite direction.

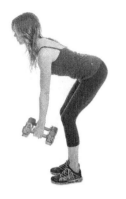 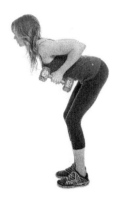

BENT-OVER DUMBBELL ROWS

A. Stand with knees bent and your torso at a sixty degree angle.

B. With the weights fully extended in your hands, bring them straight up to your chest, contracting your shoulder blades fully.

C. Slowly return to the starting position.

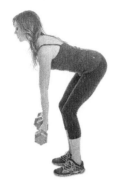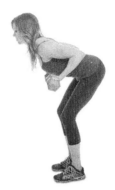

BENT-OVER DUMBBELL ROW WITH UNDERHANDED GRIP

A. Stand with knees bent and your torso at a sixty degree angle. Grasp the dumbbells with an underhand grip so your palms face up.

B. With arms fully extended, pull the weights straight up to your chest, contracting your shoulder blades fully.

C. Slowly return to the starting position.

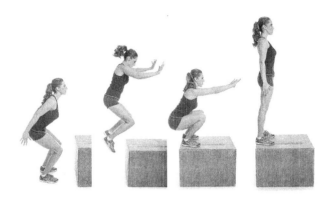

BOX JUMP

A. Stand behind a box with your feet hip-width apart or slightly wider. Engage your abs to stabilize your spine.

B. When you're ready to jump, drop quickly into a quarter squat, then extend your hips, swing your arms, and push your feet powerfully through the floor to propel yourself onto the box.

C. As you jump into the air, keep your feet level with each other and parallel with the floor. Try to land softly and quietly on the mid-foot, rolling into the heels. Do not lock your knees when landing.

D. Stand all the way up on top of the box, and extend your hips. Jump or step off the box and repeat.

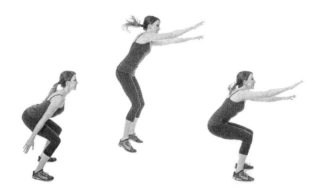

BROAD JUMP

A. Perform an air squat.

B. At the bottom position of the squat, swing your arms back and extend your knees and hips to jump powerfully forward.

C. As with a box jump, land softly and quietly on the mid-foot, rolling into the heels. You should be in a squat position. Repeat for the given number of reps.

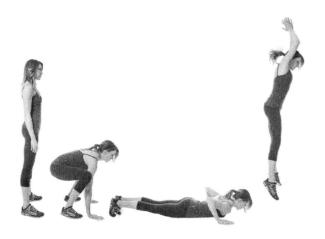

BURPEES

A. Lower your body down using proper squat form. Place hands on the ground in front of you.

B. Jump your feet back to a plank position, then quickly lower your chest to the ground.

C. Push yourself back up to a plank position and jump your feet back in toward your hands..

D. Jump back up and simultaneously clap your hands behind your head. Stand all the way, extending the hips fully before beginning your next rep.

NOTE: To modify this exercise, you may eliminate the push-up component. To further modify for beginners, you may also walk your feet out and back in instead of jumping them out and in.

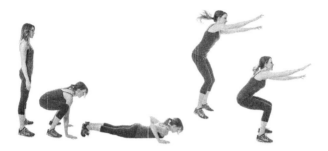

BURPEE-BROAD JUMP

A. Perform a burpee, but instead of jumping straight up, jump forward in a broad jump position.

B. Land softly in a squat position and perform another burpee.

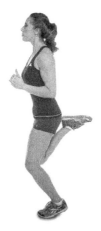

BUTT-KICKS

A. Begin by jogging normally, either in place or traveling for a short distance.

B. Then begin raising your heels up toward your bottom as you jog, using rapid, forceful movements. Again, you may either do these in place or traveling.

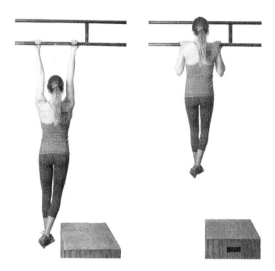

CHIN-UP

A. Step onto a sturdy chair or plyo box beneath your pull-up bar. Carefully grasp the bar with one hand, then use the other hand to help one foot into the center of the band.

B. Press down through the band to extend the leg completely. Wrap your other foot in front of foot in the band to hang from the pull-up bar.

C. Bring hands to just wider than shoulder-width, palms facing you. Keeping elbows tight to your body, pull yourself up until your chin is over the bar.

D. With control, lower yourself back down until there is just a slight bend in both elbows (don't lock them out), and repeat.

NOTE: As you become stronger, you will be able to use a smaller band until one day when you likely won't need any assistance. Make sure the band you're using provides enough of a challenge for you to help you grow stronger, and move down to a smaller band whenever possible!

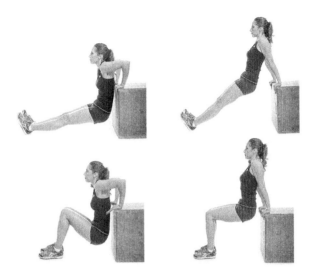

DIPS

A. Sit on the edge of a box, bench, or chair. Place hands right outside your hips, and walk your feet out in front of you so that your lower back is grazing the edge of the chair. Knees remain at a ninety-degree angle.

B. Lower your body by bending at the elbow. Elbows should not point away from your body as you lower.

C. Push heels into the floor as you straighten your arms.

NOTE: As you become stronger, walk your feet out from the ninety-degree angle until they are nearly completely straight. Keep a slight bend in the knees.

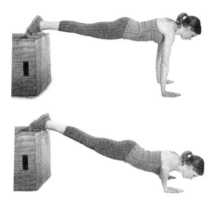

DECLINE PUSH-UP

A. Kneel on floor with plyo box, bench, or chair behind you.

B. Position hands on floor slightly wider than shoulder-width, then place feet on the elevation behind you.

C. Raise body in plank position, keeping core tight. Maintaining a neutral spine and engaged abdominals, lower yourself toward the ground by bending your arms.

D. Push through your palms to return to the starting plank position.

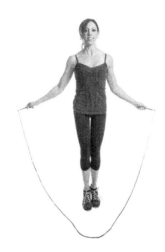

DOUBLE-UNDERS

A. First and foremost, choose a rope appropriate to your size. With the rope folded in half, it should reach up nearly to your shoulders.

B. Take one handle of the jump rope in each hand. Let the rope hang behind you so that the middle portion is hitting the back of your feet.

C. Begin my jumping rope normally. Keep elbows close to your body and wrists slightly in front of you.

D. Once you master the single-under, increase your wrist speed and jump slightly higher to pass the rope two times beneath your feet with a single jump.

NOTE: Try to use your wrists, not your arms, to rotate the rope.

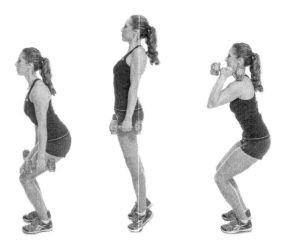

DUMBBELL HANG-CLEAN

A. Stand with your arms by your sides, hands facing inward holding a pair of dumbbells.

B. Bend both knees slightly and powerfully shrug one shoulder (this exercise is done one arm at a time., pulling the dumbbell up toward your shoulder, keeping its path as vertical as possible.

C. Aggressively drop your body under the dumbbell, rotating your elbows around the dumbbell.

D. Catch the dumbbell on the front of your shoulder (not the bone!) while moving into a quarter-squat position. Stand immediately, lower the dumbbell, and repeat for the given number of reps before repeating on the opposite side.

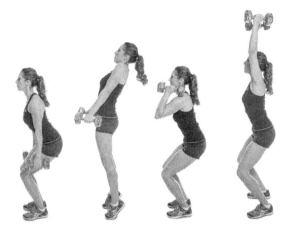

DUMBBELL HANG CLEAN AND JERK

A. Stand with your arms by your sides, hands facing inward holding a pair of dumbbells.

B. Bend both knees slightly and powerfully shrug both shoulders, pulling the dumbbells up toward your shoulders, keeping their path as vertical as possible.

C. Aggressively drop your body under the dumbbells, rotating your elbows around the dumbbells.

D. Catch the dumbbells on the front of your shoulder (not the bone!).

E. Keeping your body tight, dip down a few inches and powerfully press the dumbbells overhead, using your legs to drive the weights up.

F. Dip under the dumbbells to absorb the shock, landing with a slight bend in your knees.

G. Hold the lockout position with your arms for a second, then stand completely and lower the dumbbells to the starting position.

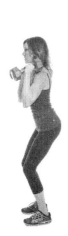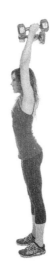

DUMBBELL PUSH-PRESS

A. Stand holding a pair of dumbbells just outside of your shoulders with arms bent and palms facing each other. Feet should be hip-width apart.

B. Dip your knees slightly then explosively push up through your legs, driving your arms upward at the same time. Make sure your biceps are by your ears in the overhead position.

C. Return the dumbbells to your shoulders and repeat.

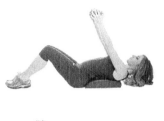

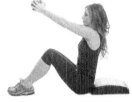

DUMBBELL SIT-UP

A. Grab your rolled-up towel or AbMat and place it above your waistband, against your tailbone.

B. Holding the end of a dumbbell in your hands with arms extended at a seventy-degree angle. Lie on your back with feet flat on the floor.

C. Keeping arms in the same position and at the same angle with feet flat remaining on the floor, lift your torso off the floor to perform the sit-up.

D. Slowly lower down one vertebra at a time to the start position.

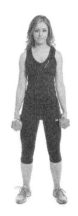
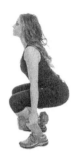

DUMBBELL SQUATS

A. With a dumbbell in each hand by either side, stand with your feet spread apart at a distance slightly wider than the shoulders. Position your feet so that your toes angle out. This angle varies from person to person, but should be about 30 degrees. Keep your weight on the heels to prevent yourself from rolling up onto the balls of your feet.

B. Keep your chest up, shoulders back, head up. This helps promote a nice, safe, intact lumbar curve.

D. Keeping dumbbells at your sides, initiate the squat with your hips pushing back, then bend your knees as you lower yourself down. Pretend there is a chair behind you that you're reaching back to sit on. Your knees should track over your feet and never jut out over them. In other words, your knees should be pointing in the same direction as your toes. If you find your knees starting to cave in, focus on pushing them out. A good way to achieve this is by imagining you are tearing the floor apart with your feet.

E. The push back up should be generated from your hamstrings and glutes. Your chest and head should remain pointing straight forward. Make sure your knees keep tracking with your toes and do not begin to buckle inwards. Also be sure and keep your lumbar curve intact (curved). Generally speaking, if you have your chest and head up, your lumbar curve will be in the correct position.

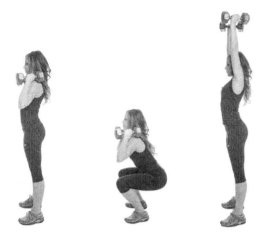

DUMBBELL THRUSTER

A. Hold a pair of dumbbells in front of your shoulders with bent elbows. Feet should be in your squat stance (see the description for "Air Squats" or "Dumbbell Squats" above.

B. Initiate the squat by pushing your hips back, then bend your knees as you lower yourself down as in a normal squat. Make sure your torso remains upright. Do not allow the dumbbells to pull you forward.

C. As your return to a standing position, explosively press the dumbbells overhead. Make sure your biceps are by your ears in the overhead position and that your legs are straight.

D. Lower the dumbbells to your shoulders and repeat for the given number of repetitions.

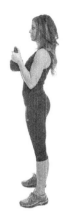
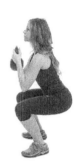

GOBLET SQUAT WITH KETTLEBELL

A. Hold a kettlebell by its horns at your chest. Stand with feet shoulder-width apart, torso upright.

B. With the kettlebell against your chest, squat down with the goal of having your elbows slide down along the inside of your knees. It's okay to have the elbows push the knees out a bit as you descend. Focus on keeping your back flat.

C. Rise out of the squat by driving through your heels.

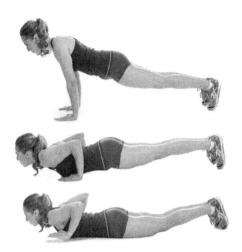

HAND-RELEASE PUSH-UP

A. Follow the steps for a "Modified" or "Traditional" push-up.

B. At the bottom position, with chest against the floor, release your hands from the floor.

C. Drive your palms in the floor to return to starting position.

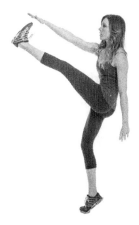

HIGH KICKS

A. Stand up straight with your kicking leg just behind your planted leg.

B. Kick your leg in front of you. Take it up as high as it will go while maintaining a straight spine as much as possible.

C. Return to the starting position, and repeat on the opposite side. You may do these in place or traveling.

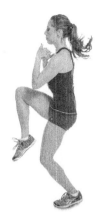

HIGH KNEES

A. Begin jogging, either in place or over a short distance.

B. Drive one knee up toward your chest and quickly return it to the ground. Follow immediately with the opposite knee.

C. Continue alternating for the given number of repetitions.

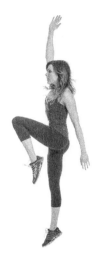

HIGH SKIPS

A. This exercise is just like a typical skip you probably did as a little girl, except the emphasis is on getting as high in the air as you can.

B. Emphasize a big arm swing and explosive knee lift on the opposite side.

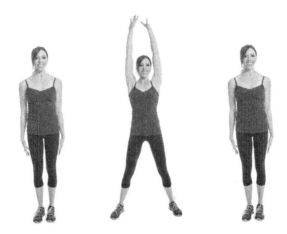

JUMPING JACKS

A. Begin by standing feet together with arms at your sides.

B. Bend your knees and jump, moving your feet apart until they are wider than shoulder-width. (You should be on the balls of your feet.) At the same time, raise your arms all the way overhead.

C. Maintain a slight bend in your knees as you jump your feet back together and return your arms to your sides. Repeat for the given number of reps.

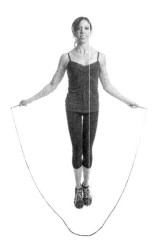

JUMP ROPE

A. First and foremost, choose a rope appropriate to your size. With the rope folded in half, it should reach up nearly to your shoulders.

B. Take one handle of the jump rope in each hand. Let the rope hang behind you so that the middle portion is hitting the back of your feet.

C. Use your hands and wrists to swing the rope over your head. Don't move your whole arm; try to keep the motion limited to your wrists.

D. As the rope comes toward the front of your feet, hop over it. Try to keep the motion in your ankles; bending your knees to jump will wear your out and make the exercise tougher!

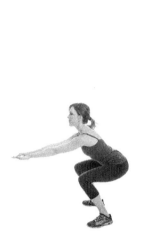
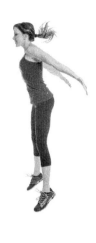

JUMP SQUATS

A. Stand with your feet spread apart at a distance slightly wider than the shoulders. Position your feet so that your toes angle out. This angle varies from person to person, but should be about 30 degrees. Keep your weight on the heels to prevent yourself from rolling up onto the balls of your feet.

B. Keep your chest up, shoulders back, head up. This helps promote a nice, safe, intact lumbar curve.

C. Place arms straight out in front of your chest. The arms should be in a comfortable position as they act as counter balance to the motion of the exercise.

D. Bend your knees as you lower yourself down. Pretend there is a chair behind you that you're reaching back to sit on. Your knees should track over your feet and never jut out over them. In other words, your knees should be pointing in the same direction as your toes. If you find your knees starting to cave in, focus on pushing them out. A good way to achieve this is by imagining you are tearing the floor apart with your feet.

E. Jump explosively to rise out of the squatting position.

F. With control, land in a squat position to complete one rep.

NOTE: Remember not to let your knees jut over your toes or let them cave inward as you jump.

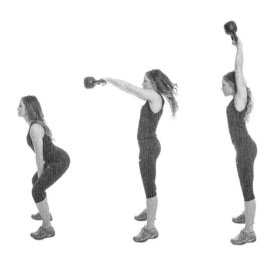

KETTLEBELL SWING

A. Hold a kettlebell (start with a light one until you're comfortable with the movement) with both hands in front of you. Stand in a squat position with feet shoulder-width apart, toes angled out slightly.

B. Lean over slightly at your waist and bend your knees as if to do a partial squat. Keep your lower back tight and arched, and keep head facing forward. Do not look down.

C. Swing the kettlebell up and overhead with an explosive hip thrust. At the top of the movement, the bottom of the kettlebell should be facing the ceiling and your biceps should be by your ears, arms fully extended.

D. Reverse the motion to return the kettlebell to the starting position between your legs, and immediately begin the next swing.

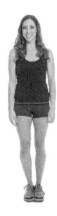
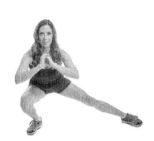

LATERAL LUNGES

A. Stand with your feet hip-width apart and make sure you have about two to three feet of space on either side of you.

B. Step sideways a comfortable distance, 2 or 3 feet, with one leg. Plant the heel of the lunging foot and keep the foot of the non-lunging leg pointed forward.

C. Sit back into the lunging leg to create a definite crease in your hip. Keep your weight in the heel.

D. Push off the heel of the lunging foot to bring feet together to the standing position. Repeat on opposite side and alternate for given number of repetitions.

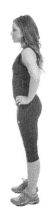
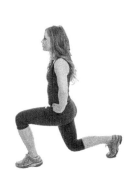

LUNGES (REVERSE)

A. Stand with feet shoulder-width apart, torso upright with arms hanging straight at your sides.

B. Take a slow, controlled lunge backward with one foot.

C. Lower your hips so that your front leg becomes parallel to the floor. At this point your right knee should be positioned directly over your ankle and your front foot should be pointing straight ahead. Your left knee should be bent at a 90-degree angle and pointing toward the floor. Your left heel should be lifted.

D. Push through both feet to straighten your legs. Bring your left foot back to meet your right in the starting position. Repeat on the other side, and continue alternating for the given number of repetitions.

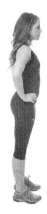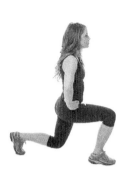

LUNGES
(WALKING AND STATIONARY)

A. Stand with feet shoulder-width apart, torso upright with arms hanging straight at your sides.

B. Take a slow, controlled lunge forward with one foot. As you lunge, lower your body and allow the lunging knee to bend until your thigh is parallel to the ground.

C. If performing a stationary lunge, push explosively off the lunging foot to return to the starting position. If performing walking lunges, push through the heel of the lunging foot to bring the back foot to meet it.

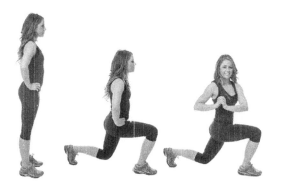

LUNGES WITH TWIST OVER LUNGING KNEE

A. Stand with feet shoulder-width apart, torso upright with arms hanging straight at your sides.

B. Take a slow, controlled lunge forward with one foot. As you lunge, lower your body and allow the lunging knee to bend until your thigh is parallel to the ground.

C. In the lunge position, bend your elbows at ninety degrees and rotate your torso in the direction of your bent knee.

D. If performing walking lunges, push through the heel of the lunging foot to bring the back foot to meet it.

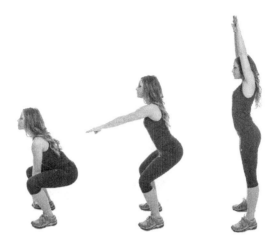

MOCK KETTLEBELL SWINGS

A. Assume an air squat stance with feet shoulder-width apart, toes angled out slightly.

B. Keeping your chest lifted and your lower back arched, reach down to the floor with your fingertips.

C. Thrust your hips forward as you stand from the squat position. Your arms should be straight, as if your hands are holding an invisible weight.

D. Swing your arms overhead until your biceps are beside your ears.

E. Squat to lower your arms back down toward the floor.

NOTE: Fully extend or "open up" your hips when you stand.

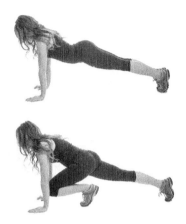

MOUNTAIN-CLIMBERS

A. Place your hands on the floor, slightly wider than shoulder-width. Step out with your feet to assume a plank position.

B. While holding your upper body in place, alternate bringing the right and left knees toward your chest.

C. Keep your hips down and increase the intensity by performing the movement faster as you feel comfortable.

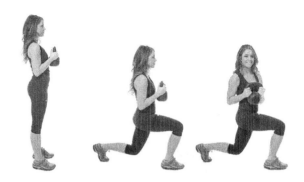

OBLIQUE TWISTS HOLDING KETTLEBELL

A. Sit on the floor holding a kettlebell at your chest. Lift your feet off the floor a few inches and cross your ankles.

B. Keeping your core tight, twist to one side, bringing the kettlebell toward your hip. Repeat on the opposite side.

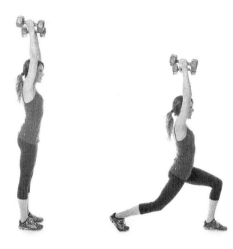

OVERHEAD WALKING LUNGES WITH DUMBBELLS

A. Hold a pair of dumbbells overhead, arms fully extended with biceps by your ears. Stand with feet shoulder-width apart.

B. Take a slow, controlled lunge forward with one foot. As you lunge, lower your body and allow the lunging knee to bend until your thigh is parallel to the ground. Keep arms strong and locked out overhead. Do not let elbows bend.

C. If performing walking lunges, push through the heel of the lunging foot to bring the back foot to meet it.

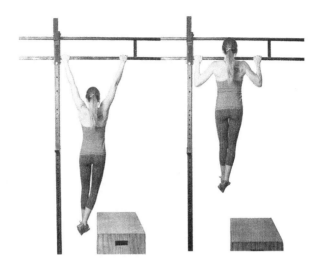

PULL-UPS

A. Hold onto the bar with a grip that's wider than shoulder-width.

B. Imagine you want to bring the bar down too your chest. This will help you pull up toward the bar until your chin is over it. Really squeeze your shoulder blades together to engage your back muscles.

C. Slowly, with control, lower yourself back down to the start position. Do not lock out your arms at the bottom, but maintain a slight bend in your elbows.

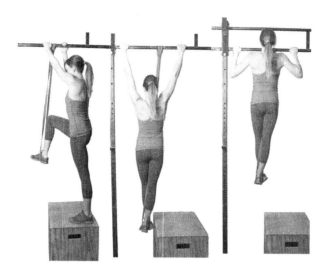

PULL-UPS WITH A RESISTANCE BAND

A. Place your foot in the resistance band so that the band centers in the middle of your shoe. Hold onto the bar with a grip that's wider than shoulder-width, and wrap the free foot in front of the foot in the band. Press down through the band so that you are essentially standing up inside of it.

B. Imagine you want to bring the bar down too your chest. This will help you pull up toward the bar until your chin is over it. Really squeeze your shoulder blades together to engage your back muscles.

C. Slowly, with control, lower yourself back down to the start position. Do not lock out your arms at the bottom, but maintain a slight bend in your elbows.

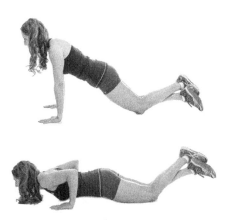

PUSH-UPS (MODIFIED)

A. Get into a hands-and-knees position on a mat or floor. Hands should be slightly wider than shoulder-width apart, fingers facing forward.

B. Keeping your core (abdominals and back) tight, slowly lower yourself in a straight line. Make sure your neck stays neutral, naturally aligned with your spine. Don't let your hips pike up in the air or your lower back sag.

C. Continue to lower yourself until your chest touches the mat or floor or, for beginners, your arms form a ninety-degree angle.

D. Keeping your spine rigid and tummy pulled in, press your hands into the floor to return to start position.

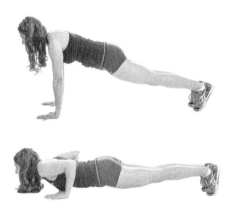

PUSH-UPS (TRADITIONAL)

A. Get into a plank position on the ground: hands and feet slightly wider than shoulder-width apart.

B. Keeping your core (abdominals and back) tight, slowly lower yourself in a straight line. Make sure your neck stays neutral, naturally aligned with your spine. Don't let your hips pike up in the air or your lower back sag.

C. Continue to lower yourself until your chest touches the mat or floor or, for beginners, your arms form a ninety-degree angle.

D. Keeping your spine rigid and abdominals pulled in, press your hands into the floor to return to start position.

NOTE: Think about exploding powerfully from the bottom position to increase the intensity to this movement.

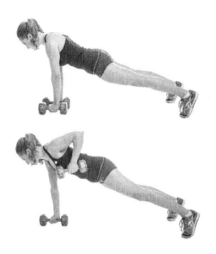

RENEGADE ROW

A. Place a pair of dumbbells side by side on the floor. Then get into a plank position with hands gripping either dumbbell, feet hip-width apart. Make sure dumbbells are about shoulder-width apart.

B. Bend your right elbow and pull the dumbbell until your elbow passes your torso. Keep the elbow tight and close to your body. Keep abdominals engaged and neck in a neutral position. Press the left dumbbell into the floor for balance.

C. Lower your arm and repeat on the opposite side.

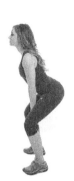 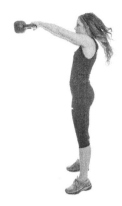

RUSSIAN KETTLEBELL SWING

A. Hold a kettlebell (start with a light one until you're comfortable with the movement) with both hands in front of you. Stand in a squat position with feet shoulder-width apart, toes angled out slightly.

B. Lean over slightly at your waist and bend your knees as if to do a partial squat. Keep your lower back tight and arched, and keep head facing forward. Do not look down.

C. Swing the kettlebell up to eye-level with an explosive hip thrust.

D. Reverse the motion to return the kettlebell to the starting position between your legs, and immediately begin the next swing.

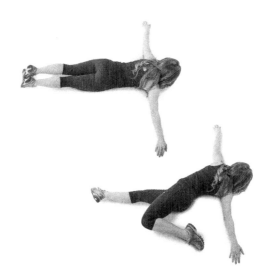

SCORPIONS

A. Lie face-down on a mat or on the floor. Stretch your arms out to either side, forming a T.

B. Lift your left leg away from the floor as far as you can, then move it to the right, crossing it over your right leg. As you do this, twist your hips to the right, allowing the left leg to touch the ground on the right side.

C. Return your left leg back to starting position and repeat the movement with your right leg.

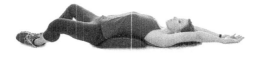

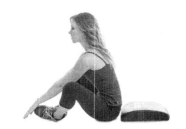

SIT-UPS

A. Grab your rolled-up towel or AbMat and place it above your waistband, against your tailbone.

B. Lie on your back with arms overhead and feet in a butterfly position (soles of feet touching).

C. Take a breath in and forcefully "throw" your arms over your body as sit up.

D. Touch your shoes as you exhale and return to a lying position, keeping the arms straight. Make sure your shoulder blades touch the floor at the bottom to achieve the full range of motion.

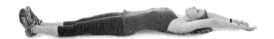

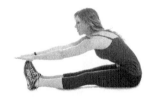

SIT-UPS TO TOE-REACHES

A. Grab your rolled-up towel or AbMat and place it above your waistband, against your tailbone.

B. Lie on your back with arms overhead and legs outstretched in front of you.

C. As with a normal sit-up, fling your arms over your body and exhale as you reach your fingertips over your legs, reaching for your toes.

D. Gently roll down, one vertebra at a time, to the start position.

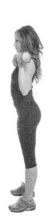
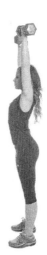

STRICT DUMBBELL PRESS

A. Stand with arms at your sides with a dumbbell in each hand. Feet should be hip-width apart.

B. Raise the dumbbells to shoulder-level, and rotate your hands so your fists face away from your body. Your elbows should be tight to your body with your forearms directly under the dumbbell handles.

C. Push the dumbbells upwards by lengthening your arms. Continue until your arms are completely extended overhead.

D. Lower the weights to start position, just until your upper arms are parallel with the floor.

NOTE: Ensure your back stays in a neutral position. Don't lean forward or backward; doing so could result in increased pressure on the spine which may lead to injury.

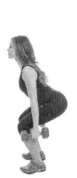 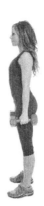

SUITCASE DEADLIFT

A. Hold one dumbbell to the side of your body. Feet are hip-width apart.

B. With shoulders back, chest lifted, and lower back in a natural arch, begin lowering your body by pushing your hips back. Then bend your knees and continue moving your rear back while maintaining the arch in your lower back.

C. The dumbbell should be lowering in a straight path in line with your shoulder blade. When you lose the natural curve in your spine and begin to round your back, stop lowering and reverse the motion.

D. To initiate the lift, use your glute muscles to powerfully thrust your hips forward. Focus on keeping your torso level and not leaning or twisting toward the dumbbell.

NOTE: As your flexibility and mobility increases, you can lower the dumbbell more and more until you can touch the floor. At that point, you can try beginning the movement from the floor.

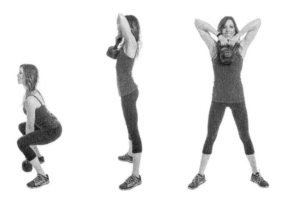

SUMO DEADLIFT HIGH PULL

A. Stand with feet slightly wider than your squat stance. The kettlebell should be in line with the balls of your feet on the ground.

B. Drop your hips and keep arms straight to grab onto the kettlebell.

C. Keeping your lower back arched and tight and chest up, use power from your legs and hips to drive the kettlebell to a top position right under your chin. Your elbows should be high, as if to form a "V" shape around your face.

D. Release your arms, bend your knees, and keep your chest high and facing forward to return to the starting position.

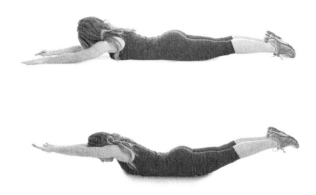

SUPERMAN

A. Lie face down on a soft surface with arms extended overhead. Keep your neck in a neutral position.

B. Keeping your arms and legs straight (not locked. and torso stationary, lift your arms and legs towards the ceiling as if to form a "U" with your body.

C. Hold arms and legs a few inches off the floor for 1 to 2 seconds and gently lower.

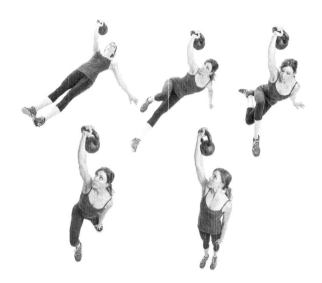

TURKISH GET-UP WITH KETTLEBELL

A. Lie on your back with your head beside the kettlebell, on the right. Grab the kettlebell's handle with your hand. Press the kettlebell straight up by locking out your arm.

B. Pull your right shoulder toward hip slightly by contracting the muscles along the side of your back and abdominals.

C. Sit up with some assistance of left arm.

D. Bend your right leg so the right foot is placed on the floor close to your hip while leaning on the extended left arm.

E. Pull the left leg back between right leg and left arm, and position forefoot and knee on floor behind right foot and left hand.

F. Position torso upright, and stand. Simply set the kettlebell down and repeat on the left side.

NOTE: Make sure you keep the wrist supporting the kettlebell straight. Never take your eyes off that kettlebell or allow your arm to loosen. Keep it tight!

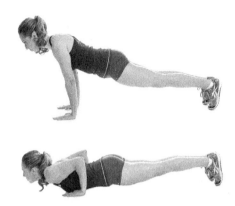

TRICEP PUSH-UP

A. Assume either a traditional or modified push-up position on the floor.

B. Bring your hands directly under your shoulders.

C. Lower your chest to the floor while keeping your upper arms parallel to your sides and your elbows pointing straight back.

D. Push back up through the heels of your hands to the starting position.

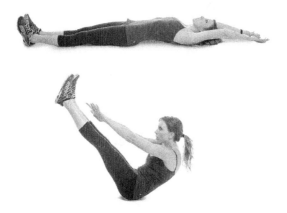

V-UP

A. Lie on your back with hands on the floor over your head.

B. Keeping knees straight and , simultaneously raise your legs and torso, reaching your hands towards your feet as you squeeze your abdominals.

C. Return gently to the starting position.

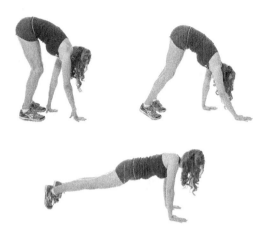

WALK OUT/WALK IN

A. Begin in a standing position. Bend over to touch your toes and walk your hands out until you are in a plank position.

B. Walk the hands back in to your feet keeping legs as straight as possible, and repeat for the given number of repetitions.

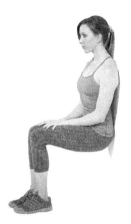

WALL SIT

A. Lean your back against a wall, leaving about eighteen inches to two feet between you and the wall.

B. Slide your body down the wall, as if trying to sit in an invisible chair. Make sure thighs are parallel to the floor. Do not slide down or raise up to make it easier!

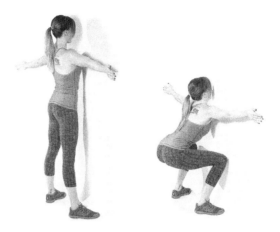

WALL SQUATS

A. Stand facing a wall, leaving just a few inches between you and the wall. Assume a squat position with shoulder-width apart, toes angled out slightly.

B. Spread arms out to either side, then squat down until thighs are parallel to the ground.

C. After a few reps, move even closer to the wall until nose and toes are against it. When you get comfortable squatting to parallel, try squatting even deeper until your hip crease is below your knees.

APPENDIX B
THE STRETCHES

Be sure to take time (5 to 10 minutes) to stretch at the end of every workout, focusing on the muscles most emphasized that day, as well as any areas that feel particularly tight or sore.

Stretching improves circulation, increases flexibility, helps maximize the range of motion in your joints, and reduces soreness and stress! Each stretch should be held between fifteen and thirty seconds and should feel good. If it becomes painful, ease up a bit, breathe deep, and go slower.

BACK EXTENSION

A. Lie on your stomach.

B. Prop yourself up on your elbows, extending your back.

C. Begin straightening your elbows until a gentle stretch is felt.

CALVES STRETCH

A. Place both hands on wall with arms extended.

B. Lean against wall with one leg bent forward and other leg extended back with knee straight and foot positioned directly forward.

C. Press rear heel into the floor and move hips slightly forward.

D. Hold and repeat on other leg.

CHEST AND SHOULDERS

A. Standing, interlock fingers behind your back, arms straight.

B. Keeping hands together, lift them as high as you comfortably can.

C. Hold for at least fifteen seconds.

HIP/GLUTE

A. Cross your left foot over right knee.

B. Grasp hands behind right thigh and gently pull thigh towards you, keeping the body relaxed.

C. Hold for at least fifteen seconds before switching sides.

INNER THIGH

A. Sit on the floor with feet pressed together.

B. Keep abs pulled in as you lean forward.

C. Keep leaning until you feel a nice stretch in your inner thighs.

LYING HAMSTRING STRETCH

A. Lie on the floor with your knees bent.

B. Straighten one leg up towards the ceiling and slowly pull it towards you, clasping your hands behind the thigh, calf, or ankle—whichever is most comfy.

C. Keep knee slightly bent. Hold for at least fifteen seconds before switching sides.

LYING QUAD STRETCH

A. Lie on your side and grasp the ankle.

B. Gently pull then ankle toward your butt, keeping your hips stable.

ONE-ARM CHEST STRETCH

A. Stand against the wall. While facing the wall, raise your right hand out to your side at chest-height, palm against the wall.

B. Turn your body toward the left, away from the wall and your extended arm, until you feel a stretch.

C. Hold and switch sides.

SEATED HAMSTRING STRETCH

A. Sit on the floor and extend one leg out straight.

B. Bend the other leg at the knee and position the sole of that foot against your opposite inner thigh.

C. Extend your arms and reach forward over the straight leg by bending at the waist as far as possible.

D. Hold and switch legs.

SPINE TWIST

A. Lie on the floor and place your right foot on left knee.

B. Using your left hand, gently pull your right knee towards the floor, twisting your spine, keeping hips and shoulders on the floor, left arm straight out.

C. Hold for at least fifteen seconds before switching sides.

STANDING QUAD STRETCH

A. Grab a stationary object, like a chair, for balance with one hand.

B. Use the opposite hand to grasp the leg around the ankle, lifting it towards the buttocks.

C. Keep your back straight.

D. Hold and switch legs.

TRICEPS

A. Standing, bend your right elbow behind your head and use your left hand to gently pull the right elbow in further until you feel a stretch in the back of your arm (tricep).

B. Hold for at least fifteen seconds before switching sides.

UPPER BACK

A. Clasp your hands together in front of your chest, arms straight.

B. Round your back towards the floor, pressing your arms away from your body to feel a stretch in your upper back.

C. Hold for at least fifteen seconds.

ACKNOWLEDGEMENTS

Above all, thank you, Abba, for being my Strength, my Shield, and my Shepherd. Every burden you lift off my shoulders. Every weapon formed against me you destroy. Every time I stray from your pastures, you call after me and guide me home. Thank you for sending your Son to reconcile us all unto you, to give us heavenly citizenship and a God-glorifying purpose on this earth. Help us to be fit to live as Jesus did, Lord.

Ben Tyler, my superhero/Prince Charming/spiritual leader and best friend. I tear up just typing your name because of all the overwhelmingly wonderful, life-changing (life-bettering!) emotions and memories I associate with it. Thank you for your constant encouragement and your never-ending faith in me, from everything to mastering an Olympic lift in the gym to finishing a book at the breakfast table. You have made me fall more in love with Jesus; I see Him in you every day and frankly don't know what I ever did to deserve you. But there's a word to answer my astonishment, I think... "Grace." I love you more than yesterday, less than tomorrow...

The ladies of CrossFit 925 and beyond: Colby, Lezlee, Merrily, Rebecca, Susan, Lynda, Andrea, Ann Marie, Heidi, Colleen, Anna, Nicole, Ashley, JoLynn, Jill, Erica, Emily, and Rachel. I cannot, in one paragraph, adequately express how blessed and blown away I've been by your contributions to this book! From the bottom of my heart, thank you for sharing yours. I know it isn't easy to openly and honestly reveal to strangers what the Lord has taught you, how He's healed and strengthened you through the storms and struggles of life. But I know that these words He's written through you will not return to Him empty, but will accomplish His desires and bless the ladies He leads to them. Through blood, sweat, tears, lots of laughter and prayers, you are my sisters and fellow warriors; I thank God for the privilege of knowing each of you.

John McBrayer, the best photographer in the universe! You were a "perfect fit" for this book; your patience, professionalism, creativity, and expertise made the photo shoot an absolutely wonderful and fun experience. I look forward to working with you much more in the future!

Heidi and Emily. Thank you for engaging "Beast Mode" for our photo shoot with John. You ladies are probably the most undiva-like models there ever were! I was so blessed to work with you on these photos. I love you both!

Last but not least, to all my awesome Tweeps who helped me generate some terrific workout ideas! *@Ashleydonde, @Lauren_Rachel, @MariaisDead, @codyferrell, @mommakristi, @jennheathcock, @CFwannabe,* and *@daimanuel.* Thank you all so much!

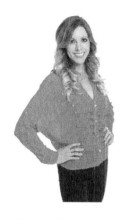

ABOUT
THE AUTHOR

Diana Anderson-Tyler earned her degree in Radio-Television-Film from the University of Texas and her personal training certification from the Cooper Clinic in Dallas, Texas. She is also a Level 1 certified CrossFit coach. She's the author of two books for women, *Miss University: A Girl's Guide to Fitness, Beauty, and Confidence* and *Fit for Faith: A Christian Woman's Guide to Total Fitness.* She has been interviewed by *The 700 Club, The Harvest Show, TCT Alive!,* and has also been a guest on several radio broadcasts, including *Changing Worldviews* with Sharon Hughes, *Rapture Ready Radio* with Matt Buff, *A Sister's Prayer* with Walda Collins, and *Take Five!* with Eddie Baiseri.

She currently writes entertainment and media-related articles for movieguide.org and contributes regularly to the health section of charismamag.com. Diana lives in San Antonio with her husband Ben. You can find Diana at *facebook.com/dianafit4faith* and on Twitter *@dianafit4faith.*

CPSIA information can be obtained at www.ICGtesting.com
Printed in the USA
LVOW05s2023151014

408908LV00032B/1276/P

9 781495 945656